DEDICATION

To our families, friends and colleagues
who have supported us in this endeavor.

ACKNOWLEDGMENT

Our thanks to all our colleagues at their respective institutions for their help and support in bringing this book to fruition. Recognition also goes to Ronnie Goldstein and Rosanne Letterese for their outstanding assistance and to the editorial staff at Professional Communications, Inc. for their creativity and understanding.

Diagnosis and Management of Pneumonia and Other Respiratory Infections

First Edition

Alan Fein, MD

Chief of Pulmonary and Critical Care Medicine
North Shore University Hospital
Professor of Medicine, State University of New York—Stony Brook

Ronald Grossman, MD

Chief of Pulmonary and Critical Care Medicine
Mt. Sinai Hospital in Toronto
Professor of Medicine, University of Toronto

David Ost, MD

Director of Bronchoscopy
North Shore University Hospital
Assistant Professor of Medicine, New York University

Bruce Farber, MD

Chief of Infectious Diseases
North Shore University Hospital
Associate Professor of Medicine, New York University

Hugh Cassiere, MD

Medical Director, Cardiac Surgical ICU
Winthrop University Hospital, Mineola, New York

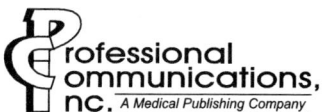

rofessional
ommunications,
nc. *A Medical Publishing Company*

Published by
Professional Communications, Inc.

ISBN: 1-884735-42-8

For orders only, please call
1-800-337-9838

Printed in the United States of America

DISCLAIMER

This text is printed on recycled paper.

TABLE OF CONTENTS

TABLES

FIGURES

1 Definition and Classification of Respiratory Tract Infection

General Information

Pneumonia has challenged clinicians since ancient times. While the lay public often believes that the problem of pneumonia has been solved by antibiotics, epidemiologists continue to report increasing mortality in specific populations. Between 1980 and 1992, the mortality rate of pneumonia increased 20%, from 25 to 30 per 100,000 population. The elderly specifically have been affected, with more than half of all deaths from infection occurring in those over age 65 years. Nine of ten deaths attributable to pneumonia occur in the elderly, while rates in children and young adults continue to decrease. While the incidence of community-acquired pneumonia (CAP) requiring hospitalization is generally 258 cases per 100,000 population, it increases to 962 cases per 100,000 population in those of age 65 years.

It has been estimated that 4 million Americans develop pneumonia annually, with 1 million hospital admissions and 10.2 million bed days. There are 20 million patient-physician interactions due to pneumonia. Inpatient care costs more than 20 times that of outpatient care, with additional expenses incurred through loss of work, catastrophic disability and prolonged recuperation. Hospital-acquired pneumonia (HAP), or nosocomial pneumonia, remains the leading cause of death due to infectious disease in inpatients, with the incidence highest in the intensive-care unit (ICU). Outside the ICU, patients with altered mental status and those who are recovering from abdominal and thoracic surgery are at highest risk. While crude mortality in patients with skin and urinary tract infections is under 5%, HAP results in death in 25% of those affected and approaches 75% in cases of virulent infections due to pathogens such as *Acinetobacter* and *Pseudomonas*.

Attributable mortality is a concept which accounts for the role of nosocomial pneumonia in adding to the likelihood that an already ill or compromised patient will die from lower respiratory tract infection; this has been estimated as one third to one half of the overall mortality. The development of pneumonia after a procedure such as cardiac surgery results in prolonged length of stay with concomitantly increased resource consumption.

It is estimated that at least 5 hospital days and approximately $1200 are added to the cost of care for each episode of respiratory infection. Once a patient is hospitalized with pneumonia, mortality takes a quantum jump from < 1% in low-risk outpatients to 14% in hospitalized patients to 30% to 40% in the critically ill pneumonia patient. It must be remembered that respiratory tract infection is an even greater problem in the developing world where prevalence of and mortality due to chronic obstructive pulmonary disease (COPD), an important pneumonia risk factor, is increasing at an even greater rate than in the United States.

Pneumonia-related challenges to the clinician include:

- Altered demographics
- New and resistant pathogens
- Economic pressure
- Diagnostic confusion and stagnation.

■ Altered Demographics

The number of elderly and immunologically impaired individuals living in the community is increasing. There remains a high reservoir of human immunodeficiency virus (HIV)-positive patients in the community along with an increasing population of transplanted patients. There is a higher incidence of respiratory tract infection and association with lower socioeconomic status and homelessness.

■ New and Resistant Pathogens

The rising problem of resistant pathogens has been recognized even in the lay press, with hospitals and businesses coming together to develop a strategy to deal with this problem. Among the most problematic are penicillin-resistant *Streptococcus pneumoniae*, methicillin-resistant *Staphylococcus aureus*, and numerous multiresistant enteric gram-negative rods, including *Pseudomonas aeruginosa* and *Acinetobacter*. Emerging pathogens such as Hantavirus and Ebola virus have become significant health risks in some parts of the world.

■ Economic Pressure

Patients, insurers and physicians are under increasing pressure to deliver quality health care at lower cost. Patients generally prefer outpatient care, with which costs are 15 to 20 times lower. The threat to quality of care brought about by limiting resources challenges clinicians to provide cost-effective care.

■ Diagnostic Confusion and Stagnation

Treatment of pneumonia today relies on empiric therapy based on epidemiologic studies of groups of patients. This will likely be a temporizing approach as more sophisticated tests based on new genetic techniques come online. These tests will allow specific identification of causative pathogens and more narrowly focused therapy, likely reducing emergence of resistant organisms linked to uncontrolled use of broad-spectrum antibiotics.

Historical Perspective

Pneumonia is a complex pathologic process which includes the accumulation of edematous fluid and inflammatory cells in the alveoli in response to proliferation of microorganisms in normally sterile lung parenchyma. The relatively defined clinical response, the inflammatory process, is the clinical illness of pneumonia.

Classifications, including typical and atypical pneumonia and, most recently, CAP and HAP classifications, have been utilized in an attempt to improve clinical relevance. Atypical pneumonia was originally applied to cases with mild symptomatology, and a more prolonged prodrome was closely associated with *Mycoplasma pneumoniae* and subsequently a variety of pathogens, including *Chlamydia* and *Legionella*. Organisms associated with this syndrome are usually associated with a more benign prognosis and offer the possibility of outpatient treatment in most cases.

In contrast, the increasing use of the hospital for treatment and the employment of immunosuppressive therapy fostered the development of a new class of patients with HAP, which has associated unique syndromes, timing of onset, prognosis and treatment. While these classifications (Table 1.1) are still relevant, the blurring of inpatient and outpatient therapy and the increasing number of immunocompromised patients in the community have reduced the utility of these paradigms.

TABLE 1.1 — PNEUMONIA CLASSIFICATION	
Community-Acquired Pneumonia	**Hospital-Acquired Pneumonia**

• Acquired at any time
• Lobar/bronchopneumonia
• Typical/atypical pathogens
	• Commonly ventilator associated
	• Early onset: < 4 d
	  – Community pathogens
	• Late onset: > 4 d
	  – Hospital pathogens

Community-Acquired Pneumonia

Lower respiratory tract infections acquired out of the hospital are labeled "community acquired." Traditionally, typical pneumonia referred to the constellation of signs and symptoms of acute onset associated with *S pneumoniae*, *Haemophilus influenzae*, *S aureus* and other gram-negative and anaerobic bacteria. Atypical pneumonia referred to the more subacute prodrome associated with *M pneumoniae*, *Chlamydia* pneumonia (also known as *Chlamydophila*), and occasionally *Legionella* species. There is, however, significant variability in the definition applied to pneumonia as assessed in a recent review. Significant overlap exists such that utilization of clinical examination to determine microbial cause of pneumonia has not been possible.

The greatest challenge to the clinician is differentiating pneumonia from upper respiratory tract infection and other conditions (ie, pulmonary embolism, congestive heart failure) which may share clinical features. In a recent meta-analysis, few clinical signs were reliably predictive of pneumonia. Once pneumonia is diagnosed, it is important to stratify these patients based on risk of complications and outcome (Figure 4.1). Physician judgment and vital sign abnormalities were the best independent predictors with likelihood ratios > 2.5. With a respiratory rate < 10, a heart rate below 100 bpm and a temperature below 37.8° C (100° F), the likelihood of pneumonia was reduced by 80%. Reproducibility of physical findings was poor. There are no uniformly established diagnostic criteria, and the expression of pneumonia even due to the same organism varies considerably depending on the age and immunocompetence of the host.

■ **Symptoms and Signs**

Signs and symptoms of CAP include:
- Fever present in younger individuals (37.8° C [100° F]); less common in patients older than 76 years
- Increased sputum production or change in color with associated cough
- Less sensitive criteria include:
  - Pleuritic chest pain
  - Dyspnea
  - Altered mentation, especially in the elderly
  - Increased or decreased white blood cell count (< 4000 or $> 12,000$ cells/mm^3).

Signs of pulmonary consolidation may also be present, but rales are more common. Dullness to percussion, bronchial breathing and bronchoegophony are not present in 65% of inpatients and 85% of outpatients with pneumonia. Elderly patients or those with significant immune deficiency are likely to incompletely express the signs and symptoms of pneumonia.

■ **Chest Radiographs**

While consolidation, infiltration and cavitation on chest radiographs are considered the gold standard for radiologic diagnosis, there is significant lack of standardization of interpretation. Some studies have pointed out a lack of concordance of interpretation of radiologic signs. The requirement of either multiple segmental involvement or new onset of infiltration may exclude mild pneumonia or infection in those with chronic underlying lung disease such as cancer. Lobar consolidation had been classically associated with pneumococcal pneumonia (Figure 1.1), but more recently has been reported to be more common than bronchopneumonia in this condition. Diffuse interstitial infiltration has been associated with atypical pneumonia, especially *M pneumoniae* (Figure 1.2).

The clinician must be cognizant of the lack of reliability of any radiologic pattern, including lobar, interstitial or cavitary. In addition, standard chest radi-

FIGURE 1.1 — LOBAR CONSOLIDATION IN RIGHT UPPER LOBE OF PATIENT WITH PNEUMOCOCCAL PNEUMONIA

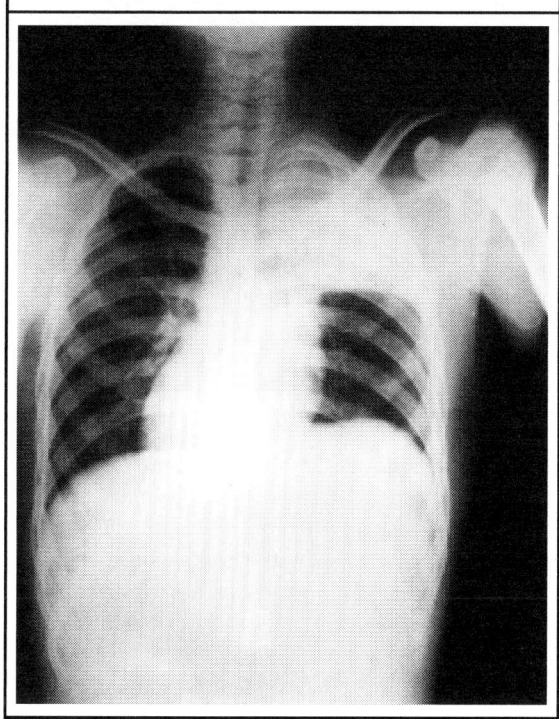

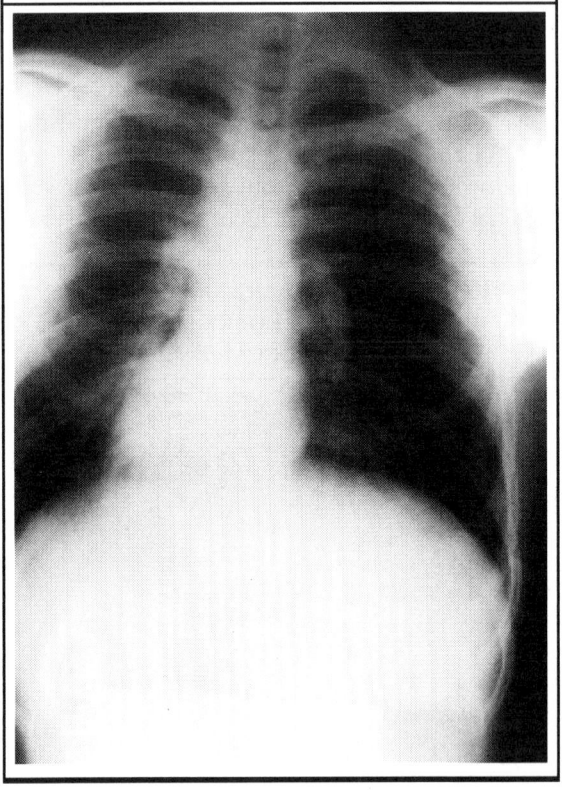

FIGURE 1.2 — CLASSIC BILATERAL INTERSTITIAL INFILTRATES SEEN IN *MYCOPLASMA* PNEUMONIA

ography may be significantly less sensitive than computerized tomography. Involvement of multiple lobes has been consistently identified as a marker of poor prognosis in CAP and should prompt consideration of admission to the ICU for observation. In the absence of altered vital signs, it is unlikely that a chest radiograph will be abnormal. Elevation of pulse, respiratory rate, and temperature or decreased blood pressure in the setting of respiratory symptoms should trigger a confirmatory chest radiograph.

Nosocomial Pneumonia

1

Nosocomial pneumonia, or HAP, is defined as an infection that develops after 48 hours of hospitalization. Ventilator-associated pneumonia (VAP) is that subset of nosocomial pneumonias that occur within the first 2 days of mechanical ventilation. Infection developing within the first 2 days of hospitalization is presumed to be acquired prior to admission. While nosocomial pneumonia is more common outside ICUs, the greatest risk is to patients requiring mechanical ventilation. In this population, the incidence is 4 to 7 per 1000 hospitalizations and develops in 25% of all ICU patients. Approximately 1% of mechanically ventilated patients will develop VAP, though the rate of acquisition declines over the time of ventilation. Gram-negative bacilli have been most often associated with VAP, accounting for the vast majority of the most common pathogens.

Nosocomial pneumonia may also be classified according to the time of onset. This classification permits the clinician to initiate treatment based on likely pathogens. Early-onset pneumonia develops within 4 days of admission and probably results from pathogens already colonizing the upper airway prior to hospitalization. Such infections usually are associated with community organisms such as pneumococcus or *H influenzae*. Pneumonia developing after 4 days of hospitalization is referred to as late-onset pneumonia and results from organisms which colonize either the gut or upper airway after admission. Organisms that replace normal endogenous flora are *P aeruginosa* and *Enterobacter* species. Criteria for diagnosis of nosocomial pneumonia include the following:

- Fever > 38° C (100.4° F)
- Leukocytosis
- Purulent tracheal secretions (usually requires positive Gram stain of > 25 leukocytes and less than 10 squamous cells per low power field)
- New or progressive infiltrate or abscess formation on chest radiograph
- Deterioration of gas exchange.

While the above criteria are sensitive, there are many causes of fever and pulmonary infiltrates which are not of infectious etiology (Table 1.2). A large body of literature has confirmed the limitation of clinical diagnosis in the cases of VAP. There has been significant variance when clinical diagnosis was compared to either histologic criteria or quantitative culture, with between 30% and 40% error rates reported, leading to significant prescription of incorrect treatment plans, including failure to:

- Diagnose pneumonia
- Recognize polymicrobial pneumonia
- Appreciate antibiotic resistance
- Eliminate unnecessary prescription of antibiotics.

TABLE 1.2 — NONINFECTIOUS CAUSES OF FEVER AND PULMONARY INFILTRATES

- Chemical aspiration without infection
- Atelectasis
- Pulmonary embolism
- Acute respiratory distress syndrome (ARDS)
- Pulmonary hemorrhage
- Lung contusion
- Infiltrative tumor
- Radiation pneumonitis
- Drug reaction
- Vasculitis
- Cardiogenic pulmonary edema

This makes the diagnosis of nosocomial pneumonia in the ICU particularly difficult. The presence of all criteria increases specificity, but it still remains below 50%. The wide differential diagnostic possibilities have led to increasing use of quantitation of bacterial cultures obtained either by aspiration or bronchoscopic sampling (protected specimen brush, bronchoalveolar lavage) to improve diagnostic accuracy.

The physician confronted with a patient with suspected pneumonia should be aware of the following caveats:

- Pneumonia may be present in patients who appear to have only an upper respiratory tract infection.
- The chest radiograph is unlikely to be abnormal in the absence of vital signs abnormalities. Pneumonia is rare when the chest radiograph is normal.
- There should be a low index of suspicion for the diagnosis of pneumonia in elderly or immunocompromised patients in whom signs and symptoms may be incompletely expressed.
- While clinical findings are unlikely to define specific microbial etiology, they are helpful in identifying potential lower respiratory tract infection and in stratifying risk so that appropriate decisions regarding pharmacotherapy and treatment setting can be made.
- Mortality in patients with pneumonia is low overall but increases dramatically in those who require hospitalization, especially in ICUs.
- Pneumonia in ventilated patients is a particularly challenging diagnostic problem. The diagnosis is often inaccurate on clinical grounds alone. Quantitative microbiologic diagnostic studies are often required.

- Ventilator-associated pneumonia adds to morbidity, mortality and resource consumption in patients who are already compromised.

SUGGESTED READINGS

Allen RM, Dunn WF, Limper AH. Diagnosing ventilator-associated pneumonia: the role of bronchoscopy. *Mayo Clin Proc.* 1994;69:962-968.

American Thoracic Society. Hospital-acquired pneumonia in adults: diagnosis, assessment of severity, initial antimicrobial therapy, and preventive strategies. A consensus statement. *Am J Respir Crit Care Med.* 1996;153:1711-1725.

Bartlett JG, Breiman RF, Mandell LA, File TM Jr. Community-acquired pneumonia in adults: guidelines for management. The Infectious Diseases Society of America. *Clin Infect Dis.* 1998;26:811-838.

Bartlett JG, Mundy LM. Community-acquired pneumonia. *N Engl J Med.* 1995;333:1618-1624.

Cassiere HA, Fein AM. Severe community-acquired pneumonia. *Curr Opin Pulm Med.* 1996;2:186-191.

Fang GD, Fine M, Orloff J, et al. New and emerging etiologies for community-acquired pneumonia with implications for therapy. A prospective multicenter study of 359 cases. *Medicine.* 1990;69:307-316.

Fein A. Treatment of community-acquired pneumonia: clinical guidelines or clinical judgment? *Semin Respir Crit Care Med.* 1996;17:237-242.

Meduri GU. Diagnosis and differential diagnosis of ventilator-associated pneumonia. *Clin Chest Med.* 1995;16:61-93.

Niederman MS, Bass JB Jr, Campbell GD, et al. Guidelines for the initial management of adults with community-acquired pneumonia: diagnosis, assessment of severity, and initial antimicrobial therapy. *Am Rev Respir Dis.* 1993;148:1418-1426.

Woodhead M. Management of pneumonia in the outpatient setting. *Semin Respir Infect.* 1998;13:8-16.

2 Pulmonary Host Defenses

Host Defenses

While utilization of recently developed clinical practice guidelines may permit a "cookbook" approach to prevention and treatment of pneumonia and bronchitis, many clinical decisions are not clear-cut and involve clinical judgment and application of physiologic and biochemical principles. Therefore, thorough grounding in normal host physiology permits a rational approach to diagnosis, treatment and prevention. This section will review normal pulmonary host-defense mechanisms and the ways in which pathology and breach of these barriers interfere with normal host-pathogen relationships, resulting in community and nosocomially acquired pneumonia. Specific aspects covered include the following (Table 2.1):

- Mechanical and structural host defenses:
  - Airway configuration
  - Cough
  - Mucociliary clearance
- Cellular host defenses:
  - Leukocytes (macrophages and neutrophils)
  - Lymphoid tissue
  - Ciliated epithelium
- Inflammatory and molecular host defenses:
  - Circulating mediators (cytokines)
  - Immunoglobulins
  - Colony-stimulating factors (CSFs)
- Humoral defenses.

TABLE 2.1 — PULMONARY HOST DEFENSES

- Mechanical and structural:
  - Cough
  - Airway branching
  - Mucociliary clearance
- Cellular:
  - Macrophages
  - Epithelial cells
  - Neutrophils
- Molecular and inflammatory:
  - Immunoglobulins: IgA, IgG
  - Cytokines
  - Colony-stimulating factors
- Humoral defenses

■ Mechanical Barriers

Mechanical barriers to pathogen invasion include the configuration of the upper airway and nasal filtering function. The continual branching of the bronchial tree, up to 20 times, into progressively smaller subdivisions results in impaction of airborne particulate matter, sedimentation and diffusion. Epithelium in the nasopharynx entraps inhaled material in a layer of mucus, where ciliary beat results in propulsion to the pharynx where it is swallowed. Ciliated epithelium is present down to the level of the respiratory bronchioles and includes at least eight different types of cells. Bacteria such as *Pseudomonas* and *Haemophilus influenzae* produce soluble products that are ciliotoxic and change mucus consistency. Changes in ciliary function occur in oxygen toxicity, following inhalation of pollutant gases like SO_2, NO_2 and cigarette smoke.

Mucus, which is composed predominantly of water, lipid, and glycoprotein (95%, 3%, 1%, respectively) with a small component mineral, has bacteriostatic and barrier functions. This glycoprotein is produced in goblet cells, serous cells and Clara cells.

Mucus is altered, structurally and functionally, by both acute and chronic inflammation. The squamous epithelium of the oropharynx interacts in a highly organized fashion with endogenous colonizing flora to prevent pathogenic bacteria from gaining a foothold.

The first stage of pathogenesis of lower respiratory tract infection is colonization of the upper airway and stomach with pathogens. This process is especially accelerated in critically ill, immunocompromised or debilitated patients. For example, gram-negative bacilli are unusual inhabitants of the oropharynx of healthy individuals and will be rapidly cleared. In contrast, during critical illness these bacterial species rapidly adhere to the oropharyngeal mucosa. This is thought to result from stasis of mucus as well as increased secretion of proteolytic enzymes, altered epithelial glycoproteins and pH. Aspiration, which occurs even in normal individuals, will be increased as changes in mental status, neurologic disease and severe illness supervene. This process will shift the balance of the host-pathogen relationship to one favoring respiratory infection.

The cough reflex, dependent on glottic closure, also ensures against prolonged infectious contamination of normally sterile lower airways. In the cough maneuver, the glottis is closed for a fraction of a second after a rapid breath inhalation. When intrathoracic pressure rises above 50 mm Hg, rapid exhalation occurs as the glottis opens. High airflow (reaching the speed of sound) progressively mobilizes mucus toward the trachea through repeated exhalations. Cough is impaired in chronic obstructive pulmonary disease (COPD), cystic fibrosis (CF), tracheotomy and intubation due to absent glottic closure. Physicians have sought to augment clearance through:

- Tracheotomy
- Supraglottic secretion removal

- The use of aerosol and parenteral medications exemplified by β-agonists, theophylline and mucolytic agents such as acetylcysteine.

Currently, there is preliminary evidence that supraglottic secretion drainage may protect against early-onset pneumonia in intubated patients.

■ Cellular Components

The cellular components of airway defenses include:
- Multiple classes of leukocytes
- Ciliated and columnar epithelium of the oro- and nasopharynx.

Alveolar macrophages are the primary line of defense of the lower airway. These cells engulf and kill bacteria such as pneumococcus and *H influenzae* when they reach the lower airway. Cell-mediated immunity is required to kill organisms such as *Mycobacterium tuberculosis*, *Legionella* and *Nocardia*, which replicate within the macrophage. If the bacterial inoculum is too large or the organism too virulent, the macrophage acts to recruit neutrophils to the site of invasion. This recruitment is the result of the initiation of the inflammatory response through complement activation, release of proinflammatory cytokines such as interleukin (IL) 8 and tumor necrosis factor (TNF), and inflammatory arachidonic acid metabolites.

Experimental studies have demonstrated a significant role for TNF in neutrophil recruitment after endotoxin challenge (lipopolysaccharide) in the lung. Similar observations suggest that TNF and IL-1 act to stimulate IL-8 production, which is a direct chemoattractant agent. This response is believed to be compartmentalized within the lung, thereby promoting local containment of bacteria without stimulating a systemic inflammatory response. Dysregulation and overexuberance of the cytokine response appear to underlie the development of the septic response. IL-10 is now recognized as a major modulator of the immune response to bacteria and serves to down-regulate the response of TNF and interferon gamma as well as other cytokines.

■ Inflammatory and Molecular Host Defenses

In addition to the role of alveolar macrophages, airway epithelia and bronchial epithelia contribute to the inflammatory process through the production of cationic, arginine-rich antimicrobial peptides called defensins, as well as the production of chemokines and IL-10. The airways of patients with CF demonstrate excessive production of inflammatory cytokines such as IL-8 which correlates with increased adherence of *Pseudomonas aeruginosa*. The anti-inflammatory agents prednisone and ibuprofen have recently been demonstrated to result in improved pulmonary function in CF patients.

Inflammatory cytokines such as IL-1 and TNF also appear to have a role in increasing adherence of *Streptococcus pneumoniae,* which binds more efficiently to type II cells and endothelium when pretreated with these inflammatory mediators. The role of platelet-activating factor receptor in this process has also been reported to enhance binding and encourage internalization of *S pneumoniae* into epithelial and endothelial cells *in vitro*.

The neutrophil is the most common leukocyte in the peripheral circulation as evidenced by the significant proportion of the bone marrow devoted to its production. This cell is essential to containment of bacterial and fungal invasion and is recruited by cytokines, such as IL-8, when alveolar macrophages are overwhelmed in the lower respiratory tract. Following active phagocytosis, fusion of phagolysosomes results in the production of potent oxidants such as hypochlorous acid.

Hypochlorous acid reacts with amines to form formidable bactericidal products. The granules of the neutrophil contain numerous proteases and acid hydrolases as well as myeloperoxidase, which contribute to its bactericidal properties. The neutrophil also actively produces defensins that act against many bacterial species and bactericidal permeability increasing protein, which acts to neutralize endotoxin. The defensins specifically interfere with the lipid membrane of the bacteria, destroying its barrier function. Reduction in circulating neutrophils below 1000/mL results in dramatically increased risk of bacterial infection of skin, mucous membrane and blood. Likewise, defective neutrophil function is seen in a variety of rare genetic diseases. In chronic granulomatous disease, there is impaired respiratory burst; in Chédiak-Steinbrinck-Higashi syndrome, lack of normal lysosomal granules is the key defect. These illnesses increase the risk of pneumonia as well as other skin and soft-tissue infections.

Recent work has sought to explore the potential of granulocyte CSF (G-CSF) as a promoter of endogenous neutrophil host defense (Table 2.2). As a class, CSFs are glycoproteins that increase the production of all blood cells and enhance their differentiation. Circulating G-CSF is increased dramatically (up to 100-fold) in patients with pneumonia and sepsis, presumably as a result of macrophage production. The response of G-CSF is not compartmentalized in the lung.

Previously used only to increase neutrophil (granulocyte) production in the bone marrow, it is now hypothesized that G-CSF may improve host survival when the non-neutropenic host is challenged by severe infection. Using G-CSF, survival has been increased in ethanol-treated mice challenged with *Klebsiella pneumoniae* and in splenectomized animals

TABLE 2.2 — GRANULOCYTE COLONY-STIMULATING FACTOR

- Increases:
  - Chemotaxis
  - Phagocytosis
  - Adhesion molecule expression
  - Respiratory burst activity
  - Bacterial and fungal killing
  - Cell life through effects on apoptosis
  - Stimulation of progenitor forms in bone marrow
  - Neutrophil antibiotic uptake

infected with *S pneumoniae*. Clinical trials in community-acquired and severe pneumonia complicated by sepsis have been reported. These data suggest beneficial effects, especially in patients with markers of severe infection such as multilobar infiltrates on chest radiograph.

The mechanism for improved outcomes is thought to be multifactorial but includes the following:

- Increased chemotaxis and phagocytosis
- Respiratory burst and expression of adhesion molecules; longer life for the neutrophil
- Increased bacterial and fungal killing
- Increased concentration of antibiotics (eg, ciprofloxacin) in the neutrophil.

By migrating in greater numbers to the site of infection or inflammation, neutrophils become antibiotic transporters. In the case of ciprofloxacin, G-CSF increased by ten times the intracellular to extracellular gradient. Concern has been raised about the potential of the proinflammatory effects of G-CSF to promote organ injury, especially in the lung. Most animal and human studies suggest that G-CSF may modulate sepsis-induced lung injury and is not toxic in doses usually administered over the short term.

Another CSF which has potential therapeutic value is granulocyte monocyte CSF (GM-CSF). Though less well studied than the related G-CSF, benefit has been observed in *in vitro* models of *Leishmania* and *Cryptococcus*, as well in mice infected with *Pneumocystis*.

■ Humoral Defenses

Humoral defenses include multiple classes of immunoglobulins (IgA and IgG). In the upper airway, IgA predominates and may account for up to one tenth of all protein in nasal secretions. Proteolytic degradation of IgA by bacterial enzymes has been demonstrated by gram-negative bacteria, including *P aeruginosa*, *Escherichia coli*, and *Serratia* and *Proteus* species. IgG gradually becomes predominant in the lower respiratory tract.

Increased IgG in the bronchoalveolar lavage of patients with inflammatory lung disease suggests the ability to recruit immunoglobulin-secreting cells into the lower airway. IgA deficiency has been associated with the propensity to develop airway infection and bronchiectasis. Pneumonia, recurrent bronchitis, sinusitis and otitis have been associated with both total deficiency of IgG as well as with decrements in subclass concentrations (IgG2, IgG4, etc).

Airway Colonization and Bacterial Adherence

Colonization refers to the continued recovery of bacteria from sites in the body in the absence of a local or systemic inflammatory response. Colonization of the upper airway is thought to be the primary step in the development of pneumonia, though in some instances the gastrointestinal tract (particularly the stomach and the trachea) may be colonized simultaneously or sequentially with the oropharynx. Bacterial colonization is initiated shortly after birth by numerous species of bacteria whose presence is thought to prevent the establishment of pathogenic bacteria. In acute or chronic illness, patterns of colonization change. Aging and the use of antibiotics also change the balance of upper airway flora to one in which pathogenic gram-negative bacteria predominate.

While the lower airway is usually sterile, primary colonization during acute illness may occur with *P aeruginosa*. In addition, recurrent or large volume aspirations with pathogenic bacteria may eventually overwhelm the defenses of the lower airway. Chronic lower airway colonization with gram-negative bacteria (eg, *Pseudomonas* species) characterizes advancing COPD and CF. Bacterial adherence is the microphysiologic interaction between host and pathogen. In the microenvironment, changes in epithelial glycoprotein receptors, pH and mucins enhance bacterial adherence. Injury to the airway is also thought to unmask binding sites to bacterial adhesion. Degradation of IgA in the airway also promotes adherence, and it has been hypothesized that vaccination to promote IgA production might reduce adherence in chronically colonized or infected individuals.

Although alteration in a single point in the integrated host-defense apparatus may occur as in selective IgA deficiency and ciliary dysfunction, more often an acute or chronic illness interferes with multiple host-defense barriers and mechanisms. For example, in COPD, cough and mucociliary clearance are impaired. In addition, associated malnutrition damages cell-mediated immunity. Chronic colonization results in inflammation and further increases bacterial adherence and breakdown of IgA. This results in a vicious cycle of inflammation, infection and bronchial and alveolar damage (Figure 2.1).

There are numerous chronic medical illnesses associated with risk of lower respiratory infection (Table

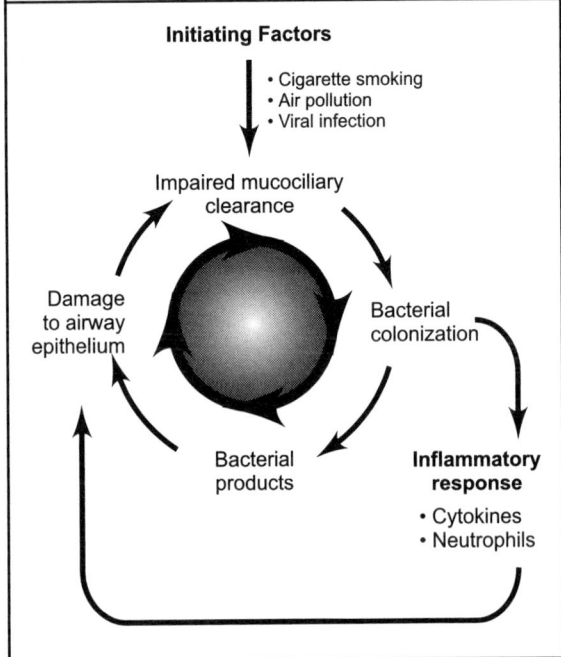

FIGURE 2.1 — SCHEMATIC DIAGRAM OF THE VICIOUS CIRCLE HYPOTHESIS IN CHRONIC BRONCHITIS

Initiating Factors

- Cigarette smoking
- Air pollution
- Viral infection

Impaired mucociliary clearance

Bacterial colonization

Damage to airway epithelium

Inflammatory response

- Cytokines
- Neutrophils

Bacterial products

2.3). Iatrogenic factors may also negatively alter host-defense balance. Among these, the use of antibiotics has been identified as a risk factor for acquisition of pneumonia with resistant organisms such as *P aeruginosa* and *Staphylococcus aureus*. The increasing pH of stomach contents observed in critical illness has been associated with progressive gastric colonization with gram-negative organisms. The use of H_2-receptor antagonists for stress-bleeding prophylaxis has also been suggested as a potential factor increasing the risk of ventilator-associated pneumonia (VAP). Patients who are mechanically ventilated have

TABLE 2.3 — MEDICAL ILLNESSES AND CONDITIONS THAT IMPACT HOST DEFENSES

- Stroke: aspiration
- Cancer:
  - Impaired humoral immunity
  - Impaired cellular immunity
- Malnutrition:
  - Impaired cellular immunity
  - Impaired secretory IgA
- Chronic obstructive pulmonary disease:
  - Cough
  - Impaired mucociliary clearance
- Congestive heart failure:
  - Impaired lymphatic drainage
  - Impaired alveolar macrophage function
- Diabetes mellitus:
  - Gram-negative colonization
  - Impaired leukocyte function
- Chronic renal disease:
  - Impaired complement
  - Impaired humoral immunity and cellular immunity
  - Impaired leukocyte function
  - Altered colonization
- Liver failure:
  - Complement deficiency
  - Impaired neutrophil activity
  - Impaired cell-mediated immunity

a risk for VAP of approximately 1% per day for the first 2 weeks after intubation (Table 2.4). This risk is clearly associated not only with concomitant immunodeficiency but also with the direct access the artificial airway provides for bacteria to the lower respiratory tract (Figure 2.2). The mucus production and epithelial damage invoked by the tube and the infectious inoculum of secretions pooled above the endotracheal cuff are also significant in the pathogenesis of pneumonia.

TABLE 2.4 — RISK FACTORS FOR VENTILATOR-ASSOCIATED PNEUMONIA

- Intubation
- Age
- High severity of illness:
  - Trauma
  - Burns
  - Chronic obstructive pulmonary disease
  - Congestive heart failure
  - Malignancy
  - Stroke
  - Sinusitis (risk higher with nasotracheal tube)
- Medical and surgical therapy:
  - Aspiration
  - Antibiotics (may protect against early VAP)
  - Corticosteroids
  - Thoracic and abdominal surgery
  - Antacids
  - Paralytic drugs

Abbreviations: VAP, ventilator-associated pneumonia.

The risk of pneumonia is also increased by the use of sedation. Though less often observed today, contamination originating in the ventilator circuit and infected condensate were previously significant sources of nosocomial pneumonia. To address this problem, reducing ventilator tubing changes from daily to every 48 hours or longer have been instituted in most hospitals. The abandonment of all routine ventilator tubing changes is a practice which evidence now can suggest reduces the incidence of pneumonia and the cost of care.

FIGURE 2.2 — PATHOGENESIS OF GRAM-NEGATIVE PNEUMONIA

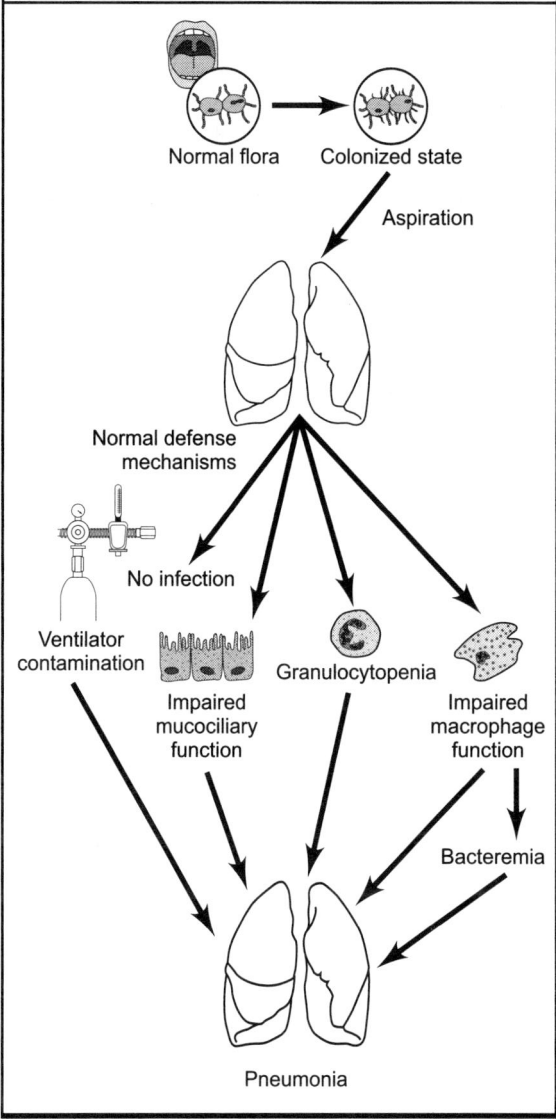

SUGGESTED READINGS

Cassiere HA, Niederman MS. New etiopathogenic concepts of ventilator-associated pneumonia. *Semin Respir Infect.* 1996;11:13-23.

Fernández-Solá J, Junqué A, Estruch R, Monforte R, Torres A, Urbano-Márquez A. High alcohol intake as a risk and prognostic factor for community-acquired pneumonia. *Arch Intern Med.* 1995;155:1649-1654.

Mason CM, Nelson S. Seminars in respiratory and critical care medicine. *Crit Care Med.* 1996;17:213-220.

Nelson S, Mason CM, Kolls J, Summer WR. Pathophysiology of pneumonia. *Clin Chest Med.* 1995;16:1-12.

Nelson S, Summer WR. Innate immunity, cytokines, and pulmonary host defense. *Infect Dis Clin North Am.* 1998;12:555-568.

Schonwetter BS, Stolzenberg ED, Zasloff MA. Epithelial antibiotics induced at sites of inflammation. *Science.* 1995;267:1645-1648.

Standiford TJ. Cytokines and pulmonary host defenses. *Curr Opin Pulm Med.* 1997;3:81-88.

Toews GB, Gross GN, Pierce AK. The relationship of inoculum size to lung bacterial clearance and phagocytic cell response in mice. *Am Rev Respir Dis.* 1979;120:559-566.

Tuomanen EI, Austrian R, Masure HR. Pathogenesis of pneumococcal infection. *N Engl J Med.* 1995;332:1280-1284.

Zeiher BG, Hornick DB. Pathogenesis of respiratory infections and host defenses. *Curr Opin Pulm Med.* 1996;2:166-173.

3

Diagnosis of Pneumonia

Although often independently classified, the diagnosis of pneumonia, acquired in the community and pneumonia acquired in the hospital share many common features. Clinical suspicion should rest on a constellation of clinical findings, which are often quite sensitive but nonspecific. In community-acquired pneumonia (CAP), patients will often present with a variety of symptoms or a "pneumonia syndrome," while in the hospital, alteration of laboratory parameters (fever, white blood cell [WBC] count, blood urea nitrogen [BUN], sputum quality and quantity) will often prompt further evaluation. The essential goals are to answer the following clinical questions:

- Does the patient have pneumonia or is the clinical picture due to some other problem?
- What is the microbial etiology of pneumonia?
- Where should the patient be treated?
- What is the best therapeutic approach to the patient's problem?

Combinations of symptoms and signs should prompt the clinician to suspect CAP (Figure 3.1). Among the most commonly seen in the previously normal host (younger, previously healthy) are:

- Cough
- Sputum production
- Fever > 38° C (100.4° F).

Less commonly seen are:

- Dyspnea
- Pleuritic chest pain
- Hemoptysis.

FIGURE 3.1 — CLINICAL APPROACH TO PNEUMONIA

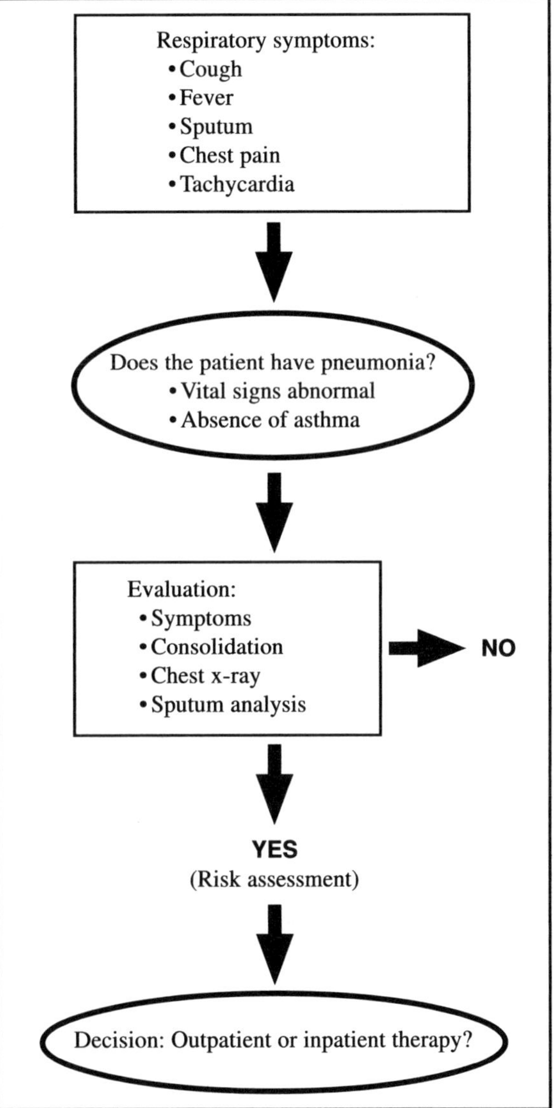

Respiratory symptoms:
- Cough
- Fever
- Sputum
- Chest pain
- Tachycardia

Does the patient have pneumonia?
- Vital signs abnormal
- Absence of asthma

Evaluation:
- Symptoms
- Consolidation
- Chest x-ray
- Sputum analysis

NO

YES
(Risk assessment)

Decision: Outpatient or inpatient therapy?

Characteristic laboratory alterations are either elevated or decreased (WBC count > 12,000 cells/mL or < 4000 cells/mL). In the elderly patient, these findings are often attenuated, and altered mental status or failure to thrive in the absence of fever or cough may be the only harbingers of pneumonia.

■ Typical Pneumonia

Typical pneumonia has been recognized for centuries as acutely producing:

- Fever (60% to 80%)
- Chills and rigors (15% to 50%)
- Chest pain (39%)
- Purulent sputum associated with intractable cough.

This syndromic grouping is observed at initial presentation in 80% of patients, regardless of age group. *Streptococcus pneumoniae* is the most commonly identified organism (> 60%) causing this syndrome.

■ Atypical Pneumonia

The original descriptions of an atypical pneumonia syndrome (Table 3.1) recognized that in somewhat younger patients, presentation is:

- More often subacute
- Associated with nonpulmonary symptoms such as:
  – Myalgias
  – Joint pains
  – Anorexia.

Atypical pneumonias were initially associated exclusively with *Mycoplasma pneumoniae* infection, but it is now recognized that a variety of other pathogens (ie, *Chlamydia pneumoniae*, *Legionella pneumophila*, *Coxiella burnetii* [Q fever]) may be causative. Patients usually seek medical attention within the first

**TABLE 3.1 — CLINICAL FEATURES
SUGGESTIVE OF ATYPICAL PNEUMONIA**

- Slow onset of pneumonia (symptoms for 3 to 4 days before patient presents to physician)
- Fever
- Chills
- Myalgia
- Headache
- Nonproductive cough
- Disparity examination of the chest and the chest radiograph (more severe)

week of illness in typical pneumonia and after a longer duration of symptoms in atypical pneumonia. This syndromic approach has been questioned by recent research, which demonstrated significant overlap in the clinical findings among pathogens traditionally associated with either syndrome; however, "pattern" recognition can suggest *Legionella* or *Mycoplasma* infection.

Additionally, in those over age 75 years, symptoms may be incompletely expressed. Fever and cough may be absent at presentation in 15% to 40% of patients. Tachypnea, tachycardia or altered mentation resulting in delirium or stupor may be the only significant findings (50% to 75% of patients). Occasionally, in the very old, pneumonia may be confused with primary neurologic disease such as stroke or intracranial bleeding. In the hospitalized patient, similar symptomatology may be the presenting picture of pneumonia.

Nosocomial pneumonia also possesses significant diagnostic challenges to the clinician. Since patients are already significantly ill, the ability to express symptoms and signs of classic infection will be diminished. The most commonly described presentation of nosocomial pneumonia includes:

- Fever

- Leukocytosis
- Purulent secretions (expectorated or sampled via the endotracheal tube in ventilated patients; findings which are sensitive but not specific).

It is essential to recognize the importance of signs and symptoms individually or as syndromic groupings. A confirmatory evaluation process should be triggered, including (Table 3.2):
- Chest radiograph
- WBC count and differential
- Chemistry profile (renal liver function tests)
- Tests of oxygenation (saturation or arterial blood gas)
- Sputum examination (Gram stain, culture)
- Blood cultures
- Pleural fluid evaluation
- Urine studies
- Serology
- Invasive procedures.

The choice among these procedures aids in the determination of whether to hospitalize and where.

Chest Radiography and Computed Tomography Scanning

The diagnosis of pneumonia may be suspected on clinical grounds but must be confirmed by chest radiography. Because many pulmonary and nonpulmonary conditions mimic the clinical findings of pneumonia, the chest radiograph permits confirmation of clinical suspicion (ie, that it is not an upper respiratory tract infection). Additionally, this test adds information that enables more accurate prognostication or leads to an alternative differential diagnosis. It has been estimated that while pneumonia or lower respiratory tract infection may be present with a normal

**TABLE 3.2 — DIAGNOSTIC APPROACH
WHEN PNEUMONIA SUSPECTED**

- All patients:
  - Chest radiography
- Outpatients:
  - Consider sputum analysis
  - Severe infection (inpatient treatment being considered):
    - Complete blood count
    - Chemistry: electrolytes, liver functions
    - Oximetry
- Inpatients:
  - Sputum evaluation:
    - Gram stain and culture
    - Acid-fast stains and mycobacterial culture
    - Tests for atypical pneumonia (*Legionella*, *Chlamydia*, *Mycoplasma*)
  - Arterial blood gases
  - Thoracentesis
  - Bronchoscopy (consider quantitative culture):
    - Critically ill
    - Respiratory failure or ventilator-dependent
    - Failure to resolve or progression

chest x-ray, this is unusual (< 5%). In fact, < 2% of pneumonia suspects who initially had a negative chest radiograph had abnormalities on subsequent radiographic examination. The suspicion of a false-negative chest radiograph should be heightened in the setting of dehydration. Case reports and animal models have suggested that dehydration will mask radiographic findings in pneumonia, which later blossoms as the patient is volume resuscitated.

Among the entities most commonly confused with pneumonia are the following:

- In the outpatient setting:
  - Upper respiratory tract infection
  - Lung cancer (2% to 4%)
- In hospitalized patients:

- Congestive heart failure (pulmonary edema)
- Pulmonary embolism
- Atelectasis or acute respiratory distress syndrome.

In the absence of vital sign abnormalities (tachypnea, tachycardia or reduced blood pressure), it is unlikely that the chest radiograph will be abnormal. Rarely, systemic vasculitides such as Wegener's granulomatosis or Churg-Strauss syndrome may confuse clinicians because of systemic symptoms and radiographic shadowing. In fact, many patients presenting with Wegener's granulomatosis are initially thought to have severe CAP. When the chest radiograph is thought to be falsely negative or when the clinical picture is uncertain, computed tomography (CT) of the chest may be extremely useful. While the chest roentgenogram should be routinely performed when pneumonia is suspected, the indications for CT of the chest are much less clear and should be reserved for complex or confusing clinical presentations or for pneumonia that either does not resolve or progresses while the patient is on appropriate antibiotic treatment.

While the chest radiograph adds to the specificity of pneumonia diagnosis, there is little evidence to support its role in differentiating among the microbial causes of lower respiratory tract infection. Numerous studies have demonstrated significant overlap between radiographic patterns of typical and atypical pneumonia. In fact, a minority of pneumococcal infections result in a lobar radiographic pattern. Both *Legionella* and *Mycoplasma* pneumonia, the classic atypical pneumonias, may present with lobar infiltration. In recent surveys, radiographic patterns were often no better than a "coin toss" in identifying specific etiologies, and interobserver reproducibility among radiologists is low. Radiologic examination may be of greater use in the diagnosis of tuberculosis. In ventilator-associated pneumonia (VAP), alveolar infiltrates with air bronchograms or progress are highly sensitive for the diagnosis of pneumonia (> 85%); specificity in this situation is unknown.

The radiographic pattern is useful in establishing prognosis and in assisting the physician in deciding the location where the patient will be best treated. Lower respiratory tract infection, which is either progressive or multilobar, identifies patients who are at higher risk for a complicated course or death. Bilateral pleural effusions in conjunction with parenchymal evidence of pneumonia are also an independent risk factor for poor outcome. These patients usually need hospitalization, and if other high-risk clinical features are present, intensive care (Table 3.3).

TABLE 3.3 — SELECTED MORTALITY RISKS

- Age > 50 y
- Tachypnea
- Hypotension
- Extremes in temperature
- Diabetes
- Cancer
- Bacteremia
- Multilobar infiltrates or radiographic progression
- Leukopenia

Adapted from: *N Engl J Med.* 1997;336:243-250.

Blood Tests: Blood Counts and Chemistry

Obtaining a WBC count is recommended when patients are being considered for inpatient therapy. While an elevated leukocyte count with left shift has often been associated with bacterial infection, it has low sensitivity and specificity. Measurement of the WBC count in outpatients should be reserved for cases in which this information will aid in the decision regarding hospitalization. Extremely high or low WBCs and bandemia are associated with poor outcome. Chemistry profiles recommended for hospitalized patients or complicated pneumonias in an outpatient setting include the following:

- Renal tests
- Liver function tests
- Electrolytes.

The role of such testing is to detect potential complications of pneumonia, including renal failure, hyponatremia and hepatitis. Elevated BUN has been identified as an independent risk factor for poor outcome.

Oxygenation Status

Arterial blood gas testing has for the most part been supplanted by the use of pulse oximetry. While routinely recommended in hospitalized patients, pulse oximetry may aid in the decision to hospitalize. If the arterial PO_2 is < 60 mm Hg or saturation < 85% on room air, patients should receive oxygen supplementation and be observed as inpatients.

Sputum Examination

When sputum is expectorated from deep within the lower respiratory tract (ie, when there is a lack of significant contamination from the upper airway tract), it provides important material for diagnostic evaluation when there is an absence of prior antibiotic therapy (Table 3.4). The former is usually determined by the cytologic criteria of < 10 squamous epithelial cells and > 25 polymophonuclear neutrophils per low-power field. When performed by an experienced examiner, Gram staining of the sputum may demonstrate characteristic lancet-shaped diplococci of pneumococ-

43

TABLE 3.4 — EVALUATION OF EXPECTORATED SPUTUM
• Good quality sputum as assessed by: – Purulence – Preferably before antibiotics started – < 10 SECs > 25 PMNs/low-power field • Transport < 2 h • Culture semiquantitatively: – 3 to 4+ growth correlates > 5 colonies in second streak
Abbreviations: SEC, squamous epithelial cells; PMN, polymophonuclear neutrophils.

cus. The Gram stain has a sensitivity > 50% and a specificity > 80% for this diagnosis. Correlation with blood cultures has been high when the specimen is of high quality. However, even studies that demonstrated strong correlation with blood culture isolates found only 25% to 50% of specimens met acceptable cytologic criteria. Perhaps this reflects the increasing frequency with which patients are treated with empiric antibiotics prior to evaluation.

In addition, atypical pathogens (mycobacteria and fungi) will not be detected by Gram staining; therefore the absence of organisms in the presence of significant WBCs on sputum examination should raise clinical suspicions. These organisms make up an increasing proportion of the pathogens encountered in CAP. Finally, there are little data indicating that improved outcomes are worth the added labor and processing expense associated with routine Gram staining. Nevertheless, this test remains a relatively simple and inexpensive means to establish a specific diagnosis, and performance should be based on the patient's ability to expectorate and the expertise of the examiner.

Sputum culture is rarely recommended in outpatients. Problems with diagnostic accuracy include contamination with upper airway flora which overgrow the true pathogen, resulting in false positives and false negatives. Additionally, problems are caused by prior use of antibiotics and inability of the patient to produce sputum derived from the lower airway. In bacteremic *S pneumoniae* infections, sputum cultures are positive less than half the time. Sputum induction is recommended in patients suspected of either tuberculosis or *Pneumocystis carinii* infection who are not spontaneously coughing. Once obtained, sputum should be cultured within 5 hours under standard semiquantitative assessment; 3 to 4+ growth correlates with > 5 colonies. Cultures are most useful for identifying *L pneumophila,* tuberculosis or endemic fungi, organisms not usually part of the upper airway flora.

Blood and Pleural Fluid

Cultures obtained from sources deep within the body which are normally sterile provide reliable and specific information regarding etiologic diagnosis. Blood cultures are reported to be positive in from 5% to 10% of patients admitted with CAP. They are generally higher in patients with pneumococcal pneumonia (25%), which indicates a worse prognosis. Although published clinical practice guidelines (American Thoracic Society and Infectious Disease Society of America) continue to recommend two blood cultures in patients hospitalized with pneumonia, the cost effectiveness of this practice has not been determined and clinical decision-making is rarely influenced by blood culture results. In addition to blood cultures, significant pleural effusions should be drained and examined by Gram stain and culture. Determination of pH and leukocyte count of pleural fluid may aid in the decision regarding the type of drainage:
- Thoracentesis
- Chest tube
- Surgical.

Routine serologic testing is not advised as the cost-benefit ratio is likely to be low. Paired samples for *Legionella* species, *Mycoplasma* or *Chlamydia* species require several weeks to increase (acute to convalescent levels) long after treatment decisions will have been made. For example, immunoglobulin M (IgM) antibodies to *C pneumoniae* take approximately 3 weeks to develop, while IgG may require 2 months. In *Legionella*, a titer > 1:256 has been considered presumptive evidence for acute infection but is present in less than 15% of documented infections. Serologic studies for viruses are also thought to be of little practical use. Cold agglutinin titers > 1:64 have a sensitivity of 30% to 60% for *Mycoplasma* and require 1 week for positivity. Thus serologic investigation aids in epidemiologic surveillance but adds little to clinical decision making.

Rapid diagnostic testing has increasingly relied on antigen detection. These techniques vary widely and include:

- Counterimmunoelectrophoresis
- Latex agglutination
- Immunofluorescence
- Enzyme-linked immunofluorescence.

Urinary antigen detection for *L pneumophila* (serogroup 1) has good sensitivity and specificity but may require 5 days to become positive. DNA amplification techniques offer promise for detection of a variety of respiratory pathogens, including pneumococcus, *Mycoplasma*, *Legionella*, *Chlamydia* and mycobacteria. Although highly sensitive, false-positive results remain problematic at the present time, and these tests have not yet had significant impact on clinical decision making in North America, although antigen detection of pneumococcus is often employed routinely in Europe.

Bronchoscopy and Related Procedures

To avoid the problems inherent with contamination of sputum specimens by upper airway flora, techniques have been developed to bypass this anatomic region and gain access to the lower respiratory tract. Transtracheal aspiration was previously used to achieve this goal but is now infrequently employed due to poor specificity and high complication rates. Bronchoscopy also can be used to obtain specimens from the lower airway but is also plagued by the problem of upper airway contamination except when tuberculosis, fungal or *Pneumocystis* infection is suspected. The use of either protected specimen brushes (PSB) or protected bronchoalveolar lavage (PBAL) allows the sample to be obtained directly from the lower airway. These techniques are now generally employed in critically ill patients. In VAP, recovery of bacteria in high concentrations (> 1000 colonies/mL for PSB or > 10,000/mL for PBAL) allows differentiation of noninfectious from infectious causes of pulmonary infiltrates.

Bronchoscopy is not recommended for routine use because of increased expense, primarily as a result of labor costs. The use of endotracheal aspirates performed by nonphysician personnel have achieved similar degrees of accuracy at lower cost. Failure to grow bacteria in an endotracheal aspiration has a high (> 90%) negative predictive value. However, the yield of quantitative culture is significantly compromised when patients have received prior antibiotics. The use of fine-needle aspiration for the diagnosis of pneumonia has been demonstrated to have diagnostic yields of 40% to 80% but carries a significant risk of pneumothorax and hemorrhage. To date, there are no studies that indicate outcome (morbidity, mortality or quality of life) is improved when invasive techniques are employed compared with empiric therapy. Bronchoscopy is of greatest value in pneumonias that progress or fail to resolve after initial empiric therapy (Table 3.5).

TABLE 3.5 — POOR RESPONSE TO THERAPY

- Inappropriate therapy:
  - Resistance (pneumococcal resistance to penicillin)
  - Organism not covered
- Unusual pathogen:
  - *Pneumocystis carinii*
  - Tuberculosis
  - Fungi
- Complications:
  - Empyema
  - Meningitis
- Complications of treatment:
  - Catheter-related infections
  - Drug fever
  - Antibiotic-induced colitis
- Noninfectious mimic:
  - Pulmonary embolus
  - Vasculitis
  - Carcinoma
  - Cardiogenic pulmonary edema

Hospitalization

The majority of patients can be treated as outpatients (> 95%). Hospitalization is mandatory in patients who are at high risk for morbidity and mortality. Additionally, social factors, including adequacy of home care, mental competence, and likelihood of compliance with therapeutic regimens, must also enter into the decision about the site of treatment.

Among the most important determinants of poor outcome are:
- Age
- Altered mental status
- Abnormal hemodynamic status
- High-risk pathogens (*Pseudomonas*)
- Cancer.

Among the best validated criteria for severity are:
- Respiratory rate > 30
- Diastolic blood pressure < 60 mm Hg
- BUN > 20
- Confusion.

Recently, the Pneumonia Patient Outcomes Research Team (PORT) developed a stratification system, which was validated in approximately 40,000 patients. Patients were divided into categories based on:
- Age
- Comorbid illness
- Physical findings
- Laboratory findings.

Those falling into category 1 or 2 (mortality < 1%) were safely treated as outpatients, while category 3 (mortality 3%) required short periods of inpatient observation. Those in category 4 (mortality 8%) and category 5 (mortality 30%) required inpatient management, the latter in intensive care. This algorithm has been endorsed by the guidelines of the Infectious Disease Society of America.

SUGGESTED READING

American Thoracic Society. Hospital-acquired pneumonia in adults: diagnosis, assessment of severity, initial antimicrobial therapy, and preventive strategies. A consensus statement. *Am J Respir Crit Care Med.* 1996;153:1711-1725.

Bartlett JG, Mundy LM. Community-acquired pneumonia. *N Engl J Med.* 1995;333:1618-1624.

Coley CM, Li YH, Medsger AR, et al. Preferences for home vs hospital care among low-risk patients with community-acquired pneumonia. *Arch Intern Med.* 1996;156:1565-1571.

Fein AM. Pneumonia in the elderly. Special diagnostic and therapeutic considerations. *Med Clin North Am.* 1994;78:1015-1033.

Fein AM. Treatment of community-acquired pneumonia: clinical guidelines or clinical judgment? *Semin Respir Crit Care Med.* 1996;17:237-242.

Halm EA, Fine MJ, Marrie TJ, et al. Time to clinical stability in patients hospitalized with community-acquired pneumonia: implications for practice guidelines. *JAMA.* 1998;279:1452-1457.

Marquette CH, Wallet F, Copin MC. Bronchoscopic invasive diagnostic techniques for the diagnosis of pneumonia. *Eur Respir Mon.* 1997;3:175-188.

Metlay JP, Kapoor WN, Fine MJ. Does this patient have community-acquired pneumonia? Diagnosing pneumonia by history and physical examination. *JAMA.* 1997;278:1440-1445.

Niederman MS, Bass JB, Campbell GD, et al. Guidelines for the initial management of adults with community-acquired pneumonia: diagnosis, assessment of severity, and initial antimicrobial therapy. *Am Rev Respir Dis.* 1993;148:1418-1426.

Pinner RW, Teutsch SM, Simonsen L, et al. Trends in infectious diseases mortality in the United States. *JAMA.* 1996;275:189-193.

Pomilla PV, Brown RB. Outpatient treatment of community-acquired pneumonia in adults. *Arch Intern Med.* 1994;154:1793-1802.

Riquelme R, Torres A, El-Ebiary M, et al. Community-acquired pneumonia in the elderly: a multivariate analysis of risk and prognostic factors. *Am J Respir Crit Care Med.* 1996;154:1450-1455.

Torres A, Dorca J, Zalacaín R. Community-acquired pneumonia in chronic obstructive pulmonary disease: a Spanish multicenter study. *Am J Respir Crit Care Med.* 1996;154:1456-1461.

Weingarten SR, Riedinger MS, Varis G, et al. Identification of low-risk hospitalized patients with pneumonia. Implications for early conversion to oral antimicrobial therapy. *Chest.* 1994;105:1109-1115.

Yu NC, Maurer JR. Community-acquired pneumonia in high-risk populations. *Semin Respir Crit Care Med.* 1996;17:255-264.

3

4 Community-Acquired Pneumonia

Epidemiology

Community-acquired pneumonia (CAP) remains a common and persistent cause of morbidity and mortality. Despite the development of multiple new antimicrobials, there is little evidence to document that either the incidence or morbidity of pneumonia has declined over the last 30 years (Table 4.1).

Unlike nosocomial pneumonia, the diagnosis of CAP is usually made more easily. Patients usually have a new infiltrate on chest radiograph, with at least two of the most common symptoms of lower respiratory tract infection, including:

- Fever
- Cough
- Sputum production
- Dyspnea
- Sweats
- Hemoptysis
- Chest pain.

Other signs and symptoms include:

- Myalgias
- Headache
- Anorexia
- Malaise
- Diarrhea
- Abdominal discomfort
- Occasionally, nausea and vomiting.

**TABLE 4.1 — OVERVIEW OF
COMMUNITY-ACQUIRED PNEUMONIA**

- Respiratory infections are the sixth leading cause of death in the United States
- Most common in the elderly, particularly during epidemics of influenza
- Major risk factors include:
  - Alcoholism
  - Smoking
  - Chronic obstructive pulmonary disease
  - Chronic congestive heart failure
  - Overcrowding
- Most pneumonia can be treated on an outpatient basis (> 80%) if carefully evaluated

A wide variety of diagnostic and therapeutic approaches has been suggested in evaluating the patient with pneumonia. Often, a brief history of the risk factors and epidemiology of the infection will narrow the focus. In addition, the duration of symptoms prior to presentation may be helpful in the differential diagnosis. Initially, one should make sure that the patient meets the diagnostic criteria. Although this is usually straightforward, caution must be used in patients with serious underlying diseases and in those who have been hospitalized in the preceding weeks. Similarly, patients who are residents of chronic-care facilities should be treated as if they have nosocomial pneumonia rather than CAP. The pattern of the infiltrate on chest radiograph may be helpful in the differential diagnosis. However, no pattern should be viewed as diagnostic for a particular pneumonia. Even the lobar infiltrates may represent atypical pneumonia.

The epidemiologic risk factors and associations are listed in Table 4.2. *Streptococcus pneumoniae* accounts for the majority of cases of pneumonia in patients over 50 years old. *Mycoplasma pneumoniae* and *Chlamydia pneumoniae* account for the majority of cases in younger adults and adolescents. It is often stated that the initial chest roentgenogram may be normal, particularly in dehydrated patients. While this can be true, one should be careful about making a diagnosis of pneumonia without some abnormality on the film. One of the major controversies of treating pneumonia concerns the issue of how aggressive the diagnostic workup should be prior to initiating antibiotics. Some feel that a highly educated guess can be made based upon age, epidemiologic risk factors and chest x-ray—that a precise microbiologic diagnosis is not necessary.

The development of the broad-spectrum quinolones and macrolides has made the empiric treatment of pneumonia easier. In addition, most studies have not demonstrated improved survival in patients when a precise microbiologic diagnosis has been made compared with those treated empirically. Finally, the yield for diagnostic workup has not been that high. Currently, expectorated sputum is diagnostic by Gram stain and culture in 40% to 50% of cases.

The counter argument that supports the need for an etiologically oriented evaluation has been outlined in a position paper by the Infectious Disease Society of America (IDSA). The rationale for establishing a precise diagnosis includes:

- To allow for organism-specific therapy
- To promote focused antibiotic selection which limits the risk of toxicity, costs and emergence of resistance
- To identify specific pathogens that may precipitate epidemiology investigations
- A precise etiologic diagnosis is valuable when the patient does not respond to therapy.

In addition, although the backbone of an etiologic diagnosis is the expectorated sputum, a number of ad-

TABLE 4.2 — ETIOLOGY OF COMMUNITY-ACQUIRED PNEUMONIA

Risk Factor for Exposure	Disease-Causing Organisms (Related Disease)
Chronic obstructive pulmonary disease	*Streptococcus pneumoniae, Haemophilus influenzae, Moraxella catarrhalis, Legionella*, gram-negative bacteria
> 60 y of age	*S pneumoniae, H influenzae*
Smoker	*H influenzae, M catarrhalis*
Alcoholism	*S pneumoniae, Klebsiella pneumoniae*, anaerobes, *Mycobacterium tuberculosis* (tuberculosis)
Influenza outbreak	*S pneumoniae, Staphylococcus aureus, H influenzae*, influenza viruses
Poor dental hygiene, loss of consciousness, seizures, esophageal disease	Anaerobes
Birds	*Chlamydia psittaci*
< 25 years of age	*Mycoplasma, Chlamydia pneumoniae*, Hantavirus
Rodent droppings	Hantavirus

Bird droppings	*Histoplasma capsulatum* (histoplasmosis)
Intravenous drug use	*S aureus*, anaerobes, *M tuberculosis* (tuberculosis), *Pneumocystis carinii* (pneumocystosis)
Farm animals	*Coxiella burnetii* (Q fever*)
Indolent presentation	*M tuberculosis* (tuberculosis), anaerobes
Animal bites	*Bacillus anthracis* (anthrax), *Francisella tularensis* (tularemia)
Travel to southwestern United States	*Coccidioides immitis* (coccidioidomycosis), *Yersinia pestis* (plague), Hantavirus
Travel to Southeast Asia	*Paragonimus westermani* (paragonimiasis)
* Q. for "query," so named because etiologic agent was unknown.	

ditional and newer technologies are now available. Some of these include:

- Sputum for acid-fast organisms in patients at risk and those with indolent presentations. Amplification methods that are reliable in patients with positive acid smears are available for this purpose.
- Tests of *Legionella* infection with urinary antigen is an easy way to screen for *Legionella pneumophila* serogroup 1. The latter accounts for 70% of all cases. Sputum culture and direct fluorescent antibody (DFA) stains on sputum are other methods whose sensitivity is dependent upon the quality of the specimen. Serology can be useful to confirm the diagnosis, but since fourfold changes in titers are needed, they are of value only in retrospect.
- Amplification of antigen nucleic acid for *Mycoplasma* and *Legionella* will be available in the near future and should be useful.
- Fungal cultures and stains of respiratory secretions will pick up *Coccidioides*, *Blastomyces*, *Cryptococcus*, *Aspergillus*, Zygomycetes (Table 4.3)
- Giemsa or Gomori methenamine silver stain is available for *Pneumocystis carinii*
- Viral cultures for influenza, adenovirus, respiratory syncytial virus (RSV); rapid antigen detection assays are now available for influenza and RSV.

These techniques should be reserved for patients in whom specific diagnosis is being considered. They are not recommended as a part of a routine workup for CAP. The IDSA does recommend that blood cultures, Gram staining and cultures of expectorated sputum be done routinely in patients admitted to the hospital.

TABLE 4.3 — FUNGAL PNEUMONIA

Normal Hosts
- *Histoplasma capulatum*
- *Coccidioides immitis*
- *Blastomyces dermatitidis*
- *Cryptococcus neoformans*

Immunosuppressed Hosts
- *Candida*
- *Aspergillus*
- Zygomycetes

4

Management

Most patients with CAP present with signs and symptoms of an acute respiratory illness. Differentiating pneumonia from sinusitis or bronchitis can often be done by physical examination, but a chest radiograph should be obtained in all patients suspected of having pneumonia. Once an infiltrate is observed, the diagnosis of pneumonia can be made if other clinical signs and symptoms are present.

The most important initial question is whether the patient will need to be admitted to the hospital or can be managed as an outpatient. The Patient Pneumonia Outcomes Research Team (PORT) has developed a scoring system that allows the severity of illness to be quantitatively measured.

Using an algorithm (Figure 4.1), the patient can be classified as to risk. The total number of points assigned to the patient increases risk of poor outcome. Patients in risk classes I, II, and III have an expected mortality < 5% and should be managed as outpatients. Patients with risk class IV and V have mortality rates of 8% to 29% and should be admitted to the hospital. Admission should be considered for:

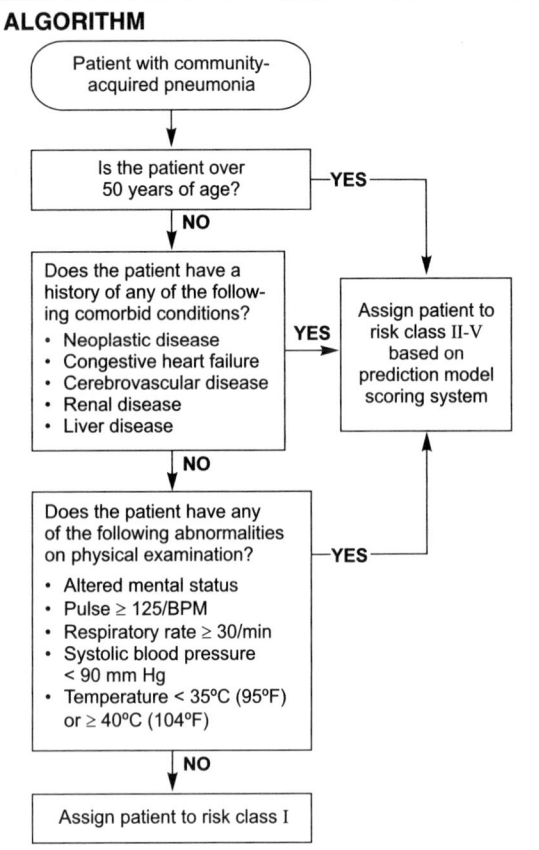

FIGURE 4.1 — PREDICTION MODEL FOR COMMUNITY-ACQUIRED PNEUMONIA PATIENT-RISK ASSESSMENT

ALGORITHM

Patient with community-acquired pneumonia

↓

Is the patient over 50 years of age? —**YES**→

NO ↓

Does the patient have a history of any of the following comorbid conditions?
- Neoplastic disease
- Congestive heart failure
- Cerebrovascular disease
- Renal disease
- Liver disease

—**YES**→ Assign patient to risk class II-V based on prediction model scoring system

NO ↓

Does the patient have any of the following abnormalities on physical examination?
- Altered mental status
- Pulse ≥ 125/BPM
- Respiratory rate ≥ 30/min
- Systolic blood pressure < 90 mm Hg
- Temperature < 35°C (95°F) or ≥ 40°C (104°F)

—**YES**→

NO ↓

Assign patient to risk class I

STRATIFICATION OF RISK SCORE

Risk	Risk Class	Based On
Low	I	Algorithm
	II	≤ 70 total points
	III	71–90 total points
Moderate	IV	91–130 total points
High	V	> 130 total points

SCORING SYSTEM

Patient Characteristics	Points Assigned*
Demographic Factors	
Age: Males	Age (in years)
Age: Females	Age (in years) –10
Nursing-home resident	+10
Comorbid Diseases	
Neoplastic disease	+30
Liver disease	+20
Congestive heart failure	+10
Cerebrovascular disease	+10
Renal disease	+10
Physical Examination Findings	
Altered mental status	+20
Pulse ≥ 125/BPM	+10
Respiratory rate ≥ 30/min	+20
Systolic blood pressure < 90 mm Hg	+20
Temperature < 35°C (95°F) or ≥ 40°C (104°F)	+15
Laboratory Findings	
Hematocrit < 30%	+30
pH < 7.35	+30
Blood urea nitrogen > 10.7 mmol/L	+20
Sodium < 130 mEq/L	+20
Glucose > 13.9 mmol/L	+10
PO_2 < 60 mm Hg[†]	+10
Pleural effusion	+10

* A risk score (total point score) for a given patient is obtained by summing the patient's age in years (age minus 10 for females) and points for each applicable patient characteristic.

† Oxygen saturation < 90% was also considered abnormal.

Prediction model for identification of patient risk for persons with community-acquired pneumonia. This model may be used to help guide the initial decision on site of care; however, its use may not be appropriate for all patients with this illness and therefore should be applied in conjunction with physician judgment.

N Engl J Med. 1997;336:243-250.

- Those with underlying immunosuppression secondary to chemotherapy
- Elderly patients
- Confused patients
- Those with impending hemodynamic or respiratory compromise.

The risk table also documents the high mortality associated with CAP in some groups. Patients with risk class V will usually require intensive care. Patients with the following characteristics should also be admitted to an intensive-care unit (ICU) and are classified as having severe pneumonia:

- Hypotension (systolic blood pressure < 90 mm Hg)
- Impending respiratory failure that may require mechanical ventilation
- Hypoxemia (PO_2 < 60 mm Hg)
- Hemodynamic instability
- Organ failure
- Deteriorating comorbid illness
- Heart failure, diabetes, chronic obstructive pulmonary disease (COPD).

In addition to the history and physical exam, particular attention should be given to determine whether the patient has any epidemiologic risk factors that may influence the initial selection of antimicrobials and diagnostic tests that need to be done. These have been reviewed in Table 4.2, but the most common include:

- COPD: *S pneumoniae*, *Haemophilus influenzae*, *Moraxella catarrhalis*, *Legionella*
- Influenzae outbreak: *S pneumoniae*, *Staphylococcus aureus*, *H influenzae*
- Poor dental hygiene, seizures: anaerobes (necrotizing pneumonia, empyema, abscess)
- Rodent droppings: Hantavirus

- Travel to the southwestern United States: coccidiomycosis.

Assuming that the patient does not have an epidemiologic risk factor, has no serious underlying disease and has not been hospitalized or been a resident of an extended-care facility, the patient's age is one of the most important factors determining which organism is most likely present. Patients over 50 years of age will most likely be infected with *S pneumoniae.* Patients that have recently been hospitalized or transferred from chronic-care facilities need to be approached as if they have a nosocomial pneumonia (see Chapter 7, *Management of Nosocomial Pneumonia*).

Although there continues to be controversy regarding the extent of the diagnostic workup that is necessary prior to initiating therapy, the approach should be individualized. In patients under the age of 35 years with an acute illness, a history, physical examination, and chest x-ray are often all that is necessary prior to the initiation of empiric therapy. In patients with a specific epidemiologic risk factor or those with severe pneumonia, additional workup should be performed.

In general, blood cultures should be done in patients who are being admitted to the hospital but are not necessary in patients who are being treated empirically as outpatients. Blood cultures are positive in about 10% of patients with pneumonia. This test has a low sensitivity but a high specificity. Sputum cultures also are of variable value, depending upon the quality of the sample and the proper handling of the specimen. The sputum should be obtained by deep cough, and the Gram stain must demonstrate an adequate number of polymorphonuclear neutrophils (PMNs) prior to proceeding with the cultures. Sputum must be transported and plated within hours of collection. Although transtracheal aspiration is often included in recommendations requiring the workup of pneumonia, it is rarely done. Sputum analysis (using both Gram stain and culture) has 50% sensitivity and 80% specificity for pneumococcal pneumonia. Sputum analysis is also useful in the diagnosis of gram-negative and staphylococcal infection. When many PMNs are seen without organisms, the likelihood of an atypical pneumonia is high.

In addition to the blood and sputum cultures, a variety of other serologic and microbiologic tests are available. More invasive tests (pleural fluid analysis and bronchoscopy) should be used depending upon:

- Epidemiologic factors present
- Severity of disease
- Response to initial antibiotic therapy.

In general, bronchoscopy to collect sputum samples is reserved for those patients unresponsive to conventional therapy or those who are critically ill or immunocompromised at the time of presentation.

Specific Types of Pneumonia

S pneumoniae (or pneumococcus) is a gram-positive coccus that grows as single cells, pairs and chains in culture. It is a classic example of an encapsulated organism, which resists phagocytosis in the absence of type-specific antibody. More than 80 serotypes exist based on specific antigens in the capsule. Immunity after infection is limited to the specific serotype. Therefore, reinfection can occur multiple times. The organisms produce disease by direct invasion of tissue, which produces an inflammatory reaction.

The pneumococcus colonizes the respiratory tract of both children and adults. It can cause a wide variety of illnesses, but the most common include otitis media, sinusitis, pneumonia, sepsis and meningitis. About 5% to 10% of healthy adults are colonized, especially during winter. The organism is spread through close contact and therefore is more common in closed and crowded areas. Host immunity is important in determining the risk of invasive disease. Although immunity to pneumococci is complex, anticapsular antibody is the most important determinant of disease. This is the major reason that vaccination is effective.

Defective antibody dramatically increases the risk of invasive pneumococcal disease. A number of clinical conditions exist that produce defective or insufficient antibody. The more common include:

- Human immunodeficiency virus infection
- Multiple myeloma
- Lupus
- Chronic leukemia
- Nephrotic syndrome
- Splenectomy.

Other factors that predispose to infection include:

- Smoking
- Influenza infection
- Chronic cardiopulmonary disease.

Typically, the onset of pneumonia is acute, with high fever, chills, cough, sputum production and other symptoms of respiratory infection. In the very elderly, the onset may be more indolent. Physical examination and radiographs suggest lobar consolidation. Although pleural effusions develop in about 20% of cases, empyema is rare. Most patients will have leukocytosis, but 10% will have leukopenia, which is considered a poor prognostic sign. A carefully obtained and examined sputum will be diagnostic by either Gram stain or culture in about one half of the patients. Blood cultures demonstrate bacteremia in a minority of cases.

For many years, penicillin was the mainstay of antimicrobial treatment of this infection. However, over the past decade, resistance to penicillin has grown dramatically. Pneumococcal resistance is classified as sensitive (minimum inhibitory concentration [MIC] < 0.1 µg/mL), intermediate (MIC 0.1 to 1.0 µg/mL), and resistant (MIC > 1 µg/mL). Most intermediate and resistant strains causing pneumonia will respond to high doses of a penicillin or cephalosporin, but failure in the treatment of meningitis is common.

In addition, high-level resistance to the cephalosporins is increasing. Equally important is the fact that penicillin-resistant strains are more likely to be resistant to other unrelated antibiotics, including the macrolides, clindamycin and trimethoprim/sulfamethoxazole. While resistance to vancomycin has not been reported and resistance to the new fluoroquinolones is extremely rare, resistance to the macrolide antibiotics is increasing and may limit the efficacy of these drugs in the treatment of patients with pneumonia (Table 4.4).

TABLE 4.4 — NEW CONCEPTS REGARDING PNEUMOCOCCAL PNEUMONIA

- Penicillin and cephalosporin resistance is common but does not predict failure in the treatment of pneumonia.
- Penicillin-resistant strains are more likely to be resistant to other antibiotics (macrolides and trimethoprim-sulfamethoxazole).
- Fluoroquinolones (grepafloxacin, levofloxacin, moxifloxacin) can all be used as primary therapy, even for penicillin-resistant strains.

■ **Legionnaires' Disease**

Legionella species cause a variable number of cases of CAP (Table 4.5). Risk factors include:

TABLE 4.5 — *LEGIONELLA*
Risk Factors   • Smoking   • Advanced age   • Immunosuppressed
Diagnosis   • Culture on selective media   • Urinary antigen (*Legionella pneumophila* genus type L)   • Serology (acute and convalescence)   • Direct fluorescent antibody testing of respiratory secretions
Therapy   • New quinolones   • Erythromycin   • Azithromycin

- Smoking
- Advanced age
- Organ transplantation.

Person-to-person transmission has not been reported. Transmission occurs through potable water in both nosocomial and community-acquired cases. Legionnaires' typically presents with:

- High fever
- Hyponatremia
- Systemic toxicity.

The sputum demonstrates PMNs but no organisms, which is also seen in other atypical pneumonias. The chest roentgenogram often demonstrates bilateral alveolar infiltrates but can mimic lobar or interstitial pneumonias. The diagnosis can be made by serology, with a fourfold rise between acute and convalescence titers (after 4 to 6 weeks), but this is of value only in retrospect. Urinary antigen is a sensitive and specific test, but can only detect *L pneumophila* serogroup 1, which accounts for about 75% of cases. The urinary antigen will not pick up other *Legionella* species or the other serotypes. Selective media can be used to culture *Legionella* from sputum and other respiratory specimens. DFA testing of sputum can also be used but has a low sensitivity and specificity. Often, therapy for Legionnaires' disease must be initiated prior to microbiologic confirmation.

Although diarrhea and hyponatremia are common, they are not at all specific for *Legionella* infections and can be seen with other pneumonias. In the past, erythromycin has been considered the drug of choice for the treatment of Legionnaires' disease. *In vitro* data on susceptibility testing do not correlate well with *in vivo* results. Recently, experience has demonstrated that a variety of other drugs are efficacious. Intravenous azithromycin is highly effective and does not have the problems of fluid overload and phlebitis associated with IV erythromycin. The newer quinolones have excellent activity and can also be used as primary therapy. Rifampin has been used as adjuvant therapy but is not used alone. Unlike other bacterial pneumonias, *Legionella* should be treated for 2 to 3 weeks to decrease the risk of relapse.

■ Other Atypical Pneumonias

Most pneumonias in young adults are due to either *C pneumoniae* or *M pneumoniae* (Table 4.6). Mycoplasma infection has been observed to increase during epidemics, which occur approximately every 3 to 4 years. These organisms can cause bronchitis, pharyngitis or pneumonia. Usually, most patients are not critically ill and can be treated as outpatients. Respiratory failure rarely occurs. Patients usually have cough, fever, sore throat and headache. Although there are clinical differences between *C pneumoniae* and *M pneumoniae*, there is so much overlap that it is impossible to tell the two apart. In addition, both or-

TABLE 4.6 — ATYPICAL PNEUMONIAS

Mycoplasma pneumoniae
- Young adults and children
- 2- to 3-week incubation period
- Associated with extrapulmonary complications
- Initial diagnosis is clinical as tests are not reliable
- Therapy with macrolides or new fluoroquinolones (grepafloxacin, levofloxacin, and moxifloxacin)

Chlamydia pneumoniae
- Most cases are mild, but can produce life-threatening pneumonia
- May cause pneumonia in association with other pathogens
- Usually considered a disease of children and young adults, but cases in the elderly are well described
- Therapy with new quinolones, macrolides, and tetracycline

ganisms are difficult to culture and the diagnosis is often not easy. Acute and convalescent titers are useful in retrospect. Cold agglutinin titers are often positive (> 1:64) with positive *Mycoplasma*, but this test is not specific. Other uncommon causes of CAP are listed in Table 4.7.

Haemophilus influenzae

H influenzae is a small, gram-negative rod (coccobacillus) that colonizes the nasopharynx like pneumococcus. There are both encapsulated and unencapsulated forms of the organism. Usually, invasive disease (ie, meningitis) is caused by the encapsulated strain type B. The unencapsulated strains can cause a variety of respiratory infections, including:

- Sinusitis
- Otitis media
- Conjunctivitis
- Bronchopneumonia.

TABLE 4.7 — UNCOMMON CAUSES OF COMMUNITY-ACQUIRED PNEUMONIA	
Disease-Causing Organism(s) (Related Disease)	**Risk Factors for Exposure**
Mycobacterium tuberculosis (tuberculosis)	Exposure to human immunodeficiency virus (HIV), foreign-born, lower socio-economic background
Pneumocystis carinii (pneumocystosis)	Undetected HIV infection
Gram-negative bacteria	Alcoholism, nursing-home resident, recent hospitalization, immunosuppression
Streptococcus pneumoniae, *Legionella*, aerobic gram-negative bacteria (severe pneumonia)	Requiring admission into intensive-care unit

The organism remains an important cause of respiratory infection in both adults and children. In addition, it can cause bronchitis without pneumonia, especially in smokers and those with chronic pulmonary disease. Like the pneumococcus, any impairment in immunoglobulin production predisposes one to *H influenzae* infection.

Most strains produce β-lactamase and therefore need to be treated with antibiotics that resist inactivation by these enzymes. The quinolones, second- and third-generation cephalosporins, trimethoprim/sulfamethoxazole and the new macrolides all have activity against these strains.

Anaerobic Pulmonary Disease

Anaerobic bacteria are normally present in the mouth. Infection of the lung follows aspiration that may be either overt or occult (Table 4.8). Often this is due to:

- Altered consciousness related to alcoholism
- Anesthesia
- Seizures
- Drug overdose
- Neurologic disease.

TABLE 4.8 — CHARACTERISTICS OF ANAEROBIC EMPYEMA
• Pleural fluid • pH < 7.1 • WBC > 10,000 cells/mm^3 • Low glucose • Culture or Gram stain demonstrating organisms
Abbreviations: WBC, white blood cell [count].

Poor dental hygiene and periodontal disease allow for the overgrowth of bacteria in the mouth and increase the risk of infection following aspiration. Clinically, the infection presents as an isolated lung abscess, necrotizing pneumonia or empyema.

Lung abscess presents with fever, malaise, foul-smelling sputum and cough. The abscess appears as a cavitary lesion on the chest radiograph, often with an air-fluid level. The air-fluid level is not usually seen with tuberculosis, which is also a well-known cause of cavitary pulmonary disease. The diagnosis usually is made clinically, as culture of sputum for anaerobic organisms is not practical or specific due to contamination from oral flora. A wide variety of anaerobic organisms can cause this infection, but β–lactamase-producing strains of *Bacteroides* are included. Empyema may occur as a primary problem or as a complication of pneumonia. It presents with a pleural effusion with the characteristics outlined in the Table 4.8.

Treatment consists of drainage, usually with a chest tube and/or surgically. All anaerobic pulmonary infections are treated with a prolonged course of antibiotics (2 to 3 weeks) (Table 4.9). A wide variety of antimicrobial agents, either alone or in combination, can be used but must have activity against these organisms. The morbidity and mortality associated with anaerobic infections is significant. In addition, often bronchoscopy is necessary to make sure that there is not an associated foreign body or tumor.

TABLE 4.9 — TREATMENT OF ANAEROBIC INFECTIONS
• Clindamycin
• β-Lactam and β-lactamase combination
• Carbapenem
• Moxifloxacin

Gram-Negative Pneumonia

Gram-negative aerobic pneumonia is usually a nosocomial infection. Colonization of the upper airway rapidly occurs in the elderly who are hospitalized or in chronic-care facilities, and often patients are admitted to the ICU. Aspiration of colonized bacteria can lead to pneumonia in the already ill patient. Community-acquired, gram-negative pneumonia is rare but is well described. It is more likely to occur in patients who have been recently hospitalized or are on steroids or immunosuppressive drugs. However, *Klebsiella* and *Pseudomonas aeruginosa* can occur in the alcoholic or debilitated elderly patient without additional risk factors. These infections are associated with a high mortality.

Viral Pneumonia

Many atypical pneumonias are falsely labeled "viral pneumonia." Epidemic and episodic adenovirus can cause pneumonia. Usually, adenovirus causes pharyngitis, adenitis and conjunctivitis more often than pneumonia. The diagnosis is made by viral culture of respiratory secretions and therapy is supportive (Table 4.10).

In the winter months, influenza is a cause of primary viral pneumonia and predisposes to secondary bacterial pneumonia. Typically, influenza has an abrupt onset after a 1- to 2-day incubation period. The illness is characterized by fever, chills, myalgia, headache and respiratory symptoms. Often the myalgia is severe and the most bothersome of the symptoms. This is due to direct viral infection of the muscles and can be complicated by myositis and myoglobinuria. Patients often appear to be toxic and may have hypoxia in the presence of a normal chest radiograph. Pneumonia occurs as a progressive interstitial process with negative bacterial sputum cultures.

TABLE 4.10 — ETIOLOGY OF VIRAL PNEUMONIA	
Risk Factor for Exposure	**Disease-Causing Organism**
Elderly, seasonal	Influenza virus
Exposure to rodents	Hantavirus
Exposure to infected case by nonimmune person	Varicella-zoster virus
Children, young adults	Adenovirus
Summer/fall seasons (pleuritis)	Coxsackievirus
Intubation, immunosuppression	Herpes simplex virus
Bone marrow transplantation	Cytomegalovirus

Influenza pneumonia can occur at any age but is more common in the elderly and is associated with a high mortality. Influenza is caused by two major antigenic types (A and B). Type A tends to cause more severe disease and is associated with most cases of viral pneumonia. In addition, influenza predisposes to bacterial pneumonia with *S pneumoniae*, *H influenzae*, and *S aureus*. *S aureus* is an uncommon cause of CAP in the absence of preceding influenza. The secondary bacterial pneumonias are more likely to present as biphasic illness that follows the initial disease by 3 to 5 days. Rapid viral antigen methods and viral cultures are available to make the diagnosis. Influenza A can be treated with amantadine and rimantadine (Table 4.11). During an epidemic, it is reasonable to initiate therapy against influenza even without microbiologic confirmation.

Vaccination of all patients over the age of 65 years and any patient with underlying cardiopulmonary disease is strongly recommended each year. Health-care workers should also receive the vaccine. The vaccine

TABLE 4.11 — THERAPY FOR VIRAL INFECTIONS	
Infection	**Therapy**
Influenza virus	Amantadine, rimantadine
Varicella-zoster virus, herpes simplex virus	Acyclovir, famciclovir, valacyclovir
Cytomegalovirus	Ganciclovir, foscarnet

is revised each year based on the most recent circulating viral isolates as antigenic shift and drift occur, making long-lasting immunity impossible.

Hantavirus is a recently described cause of viral pneumonia and lung injury. It is a collection of five viruses that are shed in the urine and stool of rodents. Aerosolization of the virus is followed by a rapidly progressive disease characterized by fever, chills, headache, nausea and vomiting. This prodrome is followed by the development of hypoxemia secondary to diffuse pulmonary injury. Circulating immunoblasts and thrombocytopenia may be seen. The diagnosis can be made by serology as high titers of immunoglobulin M (IgM) and IgG antibodies are present in the blood at the time of presentation. The history of rodent exposure is important in suspecting the diagnosis. Although the disease has been seen throughout the United States, most cases have originated in the southwestern part of the country.

Varicella is also a well-recognized cause of potentially fatal pneumonia. Varicella usually presents as a self-limited disease in children. However, in adults it tends to be more severe and is more often associated with pneumonia. Pregnant women in the third trimester and immunosuppressed hosts tend to be at higher risk for this complication. The diagnosis should be suspected in the presence of typical vesicular lesions plus pulmonary infiltrates. Treatment with an antiviral agent such as acyclovir should be initiated as soon as possible, as it is more likely to be successful if given early (Table 4.11).

Therapy

Therapy for pneumonia will be either empiric or organism specific. Even when empiric therapy is to be used, it can be individualized. The presence of epidemiologic risk factors and the severity of the disease will also influence the medications selected:

- Outpatients:
  - Macrolide (clarithromycin/azithromycin). Poor response may suggest infection with resistant pneumococcus or *Haemophilus*
  - Quinolone (grepafloxicin, levofloxacin, or moxifloxacin)
  - Consider doxycycline in young adults who do not respond to the above therapy
- Hospitalized patients:
  - β-Lactam antibiotic (cefuroxime or ceftriaxone) plus macrolide.
  - Fluoroquinolone alone (levofloxacin, moxifloxacin)
  - Use of third-generation or β-lactam/β-lactamase combination or a quinolone is encouraged in patients who are in critical-care units.
  - Suspected aspiration requires the use of primary antianaerobic drug (Table 4.11).
- Other clinical considerations:
  - Empiric anti-influenza therapy should be considered during epidemics with either amantadine or rimantadine.
  - Structural pulmonary disease or bronchiectasis should lead to consideration of anti-*Pseudomonas* therapy.

– All patients should be reevaluated within 48 to 72 hours of therapy to make certain there has not been a clinical deterioration requiring hospitalization (Table 4.12).

TABLE 4.12 — FAILURE TO IMPROVE WITHIN 48 TO 72 HOURS FOLLOWING THERAPY

Consider Alternative Diagnosis
- Cancer
- Embolus
- Hemorrhage

Obstruction
- Foreign body
- Empyema

Poor Choice of Antimicrobial
- Dose
- Drug interaction

Alternative Pathogen
- Mycobacterial
- Anaerobic
- Viral
- Fungal

4

SUGGESTED READING

Bartlett JG, Breiman RF, Mandell LA, File TM Jr. Community-acquired pneumonia in adults: guidelines for management. The Infectious Diseases Society of America. *Clin Infect Dis*. 1998;26:811-838.

Bartlett JG, Mundy LM. Community-acquired pneumonia. *N Engl J Med*. 1995;333:1618-1624.

Edelstein PH. Antimicrobial chemotherapy for Legionnaires' disease: a review. *Clin Infect Dis*. 1995;21(suppl 3):5265-5276.

Mandell GL, Bennett JE, Dolin R, eds. *Principles and Practice of Infectious Diseases*. 4th ed. New York, NY: Churchill Livingstone, Inc; 1995.

Marrie TJ. Community-acquired pneumonia: epidemiology, etiology, treatment. *Infect Dis Clin North Am*. 1998;12:723-740.

Marrie TJ, Durant H, Yates L. Community-acquired pneumonia requiring hospitalization: 5-year prospective study. *Rev Infect Dis*. 1989;11:586-599.

Sahn SA. Management of complicated parapneumonic effusions. *Am Rev Resp Dis*. 1993;148:813-817.

5

Antimicrobials Used to Treat Pneumonia

In community-acquired pneumonia (CAP), despite careful prospective studies, the etiologic agent is not found in 30% to 50% of cases. Most studies indicate a declining role for *Streptococcus pneumoniae* and the increasing importance of the atypical pathogens, including *Mycoplasma pneumoniae*, *Chlamydia pneumoniae* and *Legionella* species. This may reflect improved methods of detecting atypical pathogens. The most common pathogens among patients less than age 65 and without comorbid illnesses are:

- *M pneumoniae*
- *S pneumoniae*
- Respiratory tract viruses
- *C pneumoniae.*

β–Lactamase-mediated amoxicillin resistance can be expected in 20% to 40% of *Haemophilus influenzae* strains in North America and Europe and in almost 100% of *Moraxella catarrhalis* strains. The most common pathogens in patients who are over age 65 with comorbid illnesses are:

- *S pneumoniae*
- Respiratory tract viruses
- *H influenzae*
- *C pneumoniae*
- Aerobic gram-negative bacilli
- *Staphylococcus aureus.*

Less common pathogens include *M catarrhalis*, *Legionella* species, mycobacteria and endemic fungi.

Among patients with hospital-acquired pneumonia (HAP), aerobic gram-negative bacilli Enterobacteriaceae account for 60% to 80% of bacteria isolated, and aerobic gram-positive cocci, especially *S aureus*, for a further 20% to 30%. Other agents that are occasionally identified include *Legionella pneumophila*, viruses and fungi.

A large number of antimicrobials are available to treat pneumonia (Table 5.1). Although there is considerable overlap, different drugs and combinations are often used for CAP and HAP. The aminoglycosides, vancomycin and clindamycin all have limited and specific roles in the treatment of selected pathogens. The β-lactams (with or without β-lactamase inhibitors), cephalosporins, macrolides, fluoroquinolones and carbapenems are used as both empiric and organism-directed therapy.

β-Lactams

■ Penicillins

The basic structure of penicillin, 6-aminopenicillanic acid, is a combination of alanine and β-dimethylcysteine to form a penam nucleus. The β-lactam ring is essential for antimicrobial activity and side-chain modifications determine potency, spectrum and pharmacokinetics. Penicillins must penetrate the outer structures of the bacterial cell wall and bind to penicillin-binding proteins (PBPs). By binding to these proteins, penicillins cause termination of peptide-chain linkage and inhibit the formation of the normal peptidoglycan structure. The ability of individual drugs to penetrate the cell wall and the degree of affinity to the various PBPs determine the activity of the antibiotic. Resistance to the penicillins is related to:

- Alteration of the antibiotic target sites (PBP)
- Inactivation of the drug by enzymes produced by the bacteria (β-lactamases)
- Reduction of drug permeability into the cell.

Of the three mechanisms, production of β-lactamases which cleave the β-lactam ring is the most common and clinically relevant among *H influenzae* and *M catarrhalis*. Alteration of PBPs accounts for reduced penicillin susceptibility. Among the various enzymes, the TEM-1 and TEM-2 enzymes, which hydrolyze ampicillin and amoxicillin, are the enzymes most commonly seen in *H influenzae*. In order to counteract this problem, the penicillins have been combined with a β-lactamase inhibitor. These inhibitors bind irreversibly to and inactivate the β-lactamase and possibly potentiate the activity of the β-lactam antibiotic by binding to the PBPs. The best studied of the inhibitors is clavulanic acid, which inhibits most of the important plasmid-mediated β-lactamases.

Penicillin is adequate therapy for most cases of pneumococcal pneumonia. However, the emergence of resistance and its short half-life have markedly limited the use of penicillin G in the treatment of pneumonia. Resistance to penicillin is divided into intermediate and highly resistant strains. Intermediately resistant strains have a minimum inhibitory concentration inhibiting 90% of tested strains (MIC_{90}) of 0.1 to 1.0 g/mL, and resistant strains have an $MIC_{90} > 2$ g/mL. In the United States, up to 40% of strains demonstrate some evidence of resistance, and 5% to 15% are highly resistant. While most clinicians are uncomfortable using penicillin to treat any strain that is not fully sensitive, failures in the treatment of pneumococcal pneumonia are rarely, if ever, seen with intermediately resistant strains. Nevertheless, the growing prevalence of resistance and the narrow spectrum

TABLE 5.1 — CLASSES OF ANTIBIOTICS COMMONLY USED TO TREAT PNEUMONIA

Class	Generic Name	Trade Name	Usual Route of Administration
Cephalosporins	Cefepime	Maxipime	IV
	Cefetamet	—	PO
	Cefotaxime	Claforan	IV
	Cefpodoxime	Vantin	PO
	Cefprozil	Cefzil	PO
	Ceftazidime	Ceptaz, Fortaz, Tazicef, Tazidime	IV
	Ceftibuten	Cedax	PO
	Ceftriaxone	Rocephin	IV
	Cefuroxime	Ceftin, Kefurox, Zinacef	PO, IV
	Loracarbef	Lorabid	PO
Clindamycin	Clindamycin	Cleocin	IV, PO
β-Lactamase Inhibitors	Ampicillin/sulbactam	Unasyn	IV
	Piperacillin/tazobactam	Zosyn	IV
	Ticarcillin/clavulanate	Timentin	IV

Carbapenems	Imipenem/cilastatin	Primaxin	IM, IV
	Meropenem	Merrem	IV
Quinolones	Ciprofloxacin	Cipro	PO, IV
	Grepafloxacin	Raxar	PO
	Levofloxacin	Levaquin	PO, IV
	Moxifloxacin	Avelox	PO, IV (pending)
Macrolides	Azithromycin	Zithromax	PO, IV
	Clarithromycin	Biaxin	PO
	Dirithromycin	Dynabac	PO
	Erythromycin	Erythrocin	PO, IV
	Roxithromycin*	Rulid	PO

Abbreviations: PO, oral; IV, intravenous; IM, intramuscular.

* Not available in the United States.

5

of penicillin has markedly limited its use. In addition, its short half-life has made intravenous administration inconvenient. Penicillin must be given every 4 hours by the intravenous route or every 12 hours intramuscularly. Even if appropriate therapy is initiated early in the course of therapy, treatment failure is up to 10% to 15% of cases.

■ Aminopenicillins

The aminopenicillins are formed by the addition of an amino group to the basic structure of benzylpenicillin. Esters, condensates and analogues have essentially the same activity as the parent compound. Combining amoxicillin with clavulanic acid stabilizes the activity of the aminopenicillin against β–lactamase-producing strains of *H influenzae* and *M catarrhalis* but does not change its activity against *S pneumoniae*. Ampicillin is incompletely absorbed (30%) following oral administration and reaches a peak serum concentration of 2 to 6 mg/L 2 hours after a single 500-mg dose. Amoxicillin is 90% absorbed after oral administration and a 500-mg dose produces peak serum concentrations of about 10 mg/L within 1 hour.

Approximately 75% of the drug is excreted renally, and there is 17% to 20% protein binding. Minimal dosing adjustments are required in the presence of renal failure. Amoxicillin/clavulanic acid is well absorbed from the gastrointestinal (GI) tract. It has excellent penetration into most extravascular fluids and tissues, including lung and pleura. With the emergence of widespread resistance, amoxicillin has been relegated to second-line status for the treatment of severe infections. In respiratory tract infections, the increasing resistance of *H influenzae* to ampicillin and the recognition of *M catarrhalis* as an important pathogen (which, most of the time, is ampicillin-resistant) have led to the declining use of this agent. Amoxicillin/clavulanic acid is particularly useful when infections are due to β–lactamase-producing strains of *H influenzae* and *M catarrhalis*. Amoxicillin/clavulanic acid is available in 250-mg or 500-mg tablets, both of which contain 125 mg of clavulanic acid. The usual dose is 250 or 500 mg tid. A new formulation of 750 mg amoxicillin/125 mg clavulanic acid given twice daily is clinically equivalent to other dosage forms but with reduced diarrhea.

The parenteral equivalents of amoxicillin/clavulanic acid are broad-spectrum compounds with activity against a number of gram-negative rods and with some activity against *Pseudomonas aeruginosa* (ticarcillin/clavulanic acid [Timentin], piperacillin/tazobactam [Zosyn]). The addition of the β-lactamase inhibitor improves the activity against *S aureus*, *Escherichia coli*, *Klebsiella pneumoniae*, *Bacteroides* species, *H influenzae*, *M catarrhalis* but not against *Pseudomonas*, *Enterobacter*, *Serratia* and *Citrobacter* species. The appearance of chromosomally mediated β-lactamases that are not neutralized by these inhibitors, particularly among *Enterobacter* species, has limited their use, especially in severe nosocomial pneumonia. Side effects of these drugs include diarrhea, hypokalemia and minor antiplatelet activity. Ticarcillin and piperacillin are sodium salts and may precipitate heart failure in susceptible individuals. While ticarcillin and piperacillin have anti-pseudomonal activity, the addition of the β-lactamase inhibitor does not change this activity. These drugs are not sufficient as monotherapy for proven *Pseudomonas* infection, and an aminoglycoside or antipseudomonal fluoroquinolone (ciprofloxacin) should be added in these cases.

Cephalosporins

The cephalosporins are usually classified into four generations:

- The first-generation cephalosporins have excellent activity against gram-positive organisms, including pneumococci and staphylococci. Their role in empiric therapy is limited but may be used for organism-specific therapy.
- The second-generation cephalosporins demonstrate improved gram-negative coverage particularly against *H influenzae*.
- The third-generation cephalosporins have a more extensive gram-negative coverage but are weaker against the gram-positives, especially *S aureus*.
- The fourth-generation cephalosporins have extensive gram-negative and gram-positive coverage. These agents are commonly used in the treatment of immunocompromised patients susceptible to gram-negative infections and in very sick patients, typically nursing-home residents, with CAP.

None of these compounds has any significant activity against "atypical" pathogens. Since *C pneumoniae* and *Legionella* are intracellular pathogens and β-lactamase antibiotics do not penetrate into cells, this outcome is predictable.

The development of effective oral cephalosporins has been limited by the hydrophilic nature of these compounds. Recently, several oral cephalosporin derivatives have been developed which have an aminothiazolyl-methoxyimino side chain added to the cephem nucleus, resulting in greater activity against gram-negative organisms. These are generally divided into two groups. The prodrug esters include cefuroxime axetil, cefetamet pivoxil, and cefpodoxime proxetil, the side chains of which are hydrolysed by esterases in the gut wall, releasing the active compound into the portal blood. Ceftibuten is a third-generation agent that is absorbed intact. Loracarbef and cefprozil are two other newly released oral cephalosporin derivatives. The MIC_{90} values for all discussed cephalosporins are displayed in Table 5.2. Pharmacokinetic properties are summarized in Table 5.3.

■ Cefuroxime Axetil

Cefuroxime axetil is a prodrug oral formulation of the injectable cefuroxime sodium. The 1-(acetyloxy) ethyl ester of cefuroxime undergoes complete hydrolysis during absorption to free cefuroxime, which is the active antimicrobial. It is considerably more active than cefaclor against *S pneumoniae* (MIC_{90} 0.25 mg/L vs 4 mg/L), *H influenzae* (including β–lactamase-producing strains [MIC_{90} 0.25 mg/L vs 4 mg/L]) and *M catarrhalis* (MIC_{90} 0.25 mg/L vs 2 mg/L). Following a 500-mg oral dose, peak concentrations averaging 4.9 mg/L are observed within 2.3 hours. The elimination half-life ranges from 0.8 to 2 hours, similar to that of the injectable product. The oral bioavailability ranges from 30% to 45%, and it may be higher if the drug is given with food.

The major adverse event is GI related, with most studies reporting diarrhea in 3% to 5% of patients. Nausea, vomiting or heartburn have occurred in < 4% of patients. As with other cephalosporins, antibiotic-induced colitis has been reported with this agent. The usual dosage is 250 mg bid, but it may be increased to 500 mg bid for serious infections.

In patients with lower respiratory tract infections, cefuroxime axetil 250 or 500 mg every 12 hours has clinical and bacteriologic cure rates similar to those of cefaclor given in a dosage of 500 mg every 8 hours. Cefuroxime axetil has good activity against all major respiratory pathogens except for the "atypical" organisms such as *C pneumoniae*, *M pneumoniae* or

TABLE 5.2 — IN VITRO MIC$_{90}$ VALUES (MG/L) OF ORAL CEPHALOSPORINS AGAINST SELECTED RESPIRATORY PATHOGENS

Organism	Cefetamet	Cefpodoxime	Cefprozil	Ceftibuten	Cefuroxime	Loracarbef
Klebsiella pneumoniae	0.58	0.9	> 16.7	0.15	4	1-8
*Haemophilus influenzae**	0.57	< 0.24	6.7-12.9	< 0.11-0.22	0.25	0.5-16
*Moraxella catarrhalis**	0.79	0.63	4.5	2.6-2.9	0.25	< 0.25-8
Staphylococcus aureus	> 57	2.5	1.4	> 32	1	1-8
Streptococcus pneumoniae	0.55	< 0.05	0.23	4-8	0.25	0.5-2
Streptococcus pyogenes	< 0.22	< 0.02	0.04	0.5-2	0.5	0.12-1

Abbreviations: MIC$_{90}$, concentration inhibiting 90% of tested strains.

* β–Lactamase-producing and β–lactamase-negative strains.

TABLE 5.3 — PHARMACOKINETIC PROPERTIES OF CEPHALOSPORINS

Drug	Dose (mg)	T_{max} (h)	Protein Binding (%)	C_{max} (mg/L)	$t\frac{1}{2} B$ (h)
Cefetamet	500	3.0	22	4.1	2.3
Cefpodoxime	400	2.9	40	4.2	2.6
Cefprozil	500	3.2	42	9.6	1.4
Ceftibuten	200	1.8	63	10.9	2.5
Cefuroxime	500	2.4	33	5.6	1.5
Loracarbef	400	1.4	35	11.2	1.3

Abbreviations: T_{max}, time to maximum serum concentration; C_{max}, maximum serum concentration; $t\frac{1}{2} B$, terminal half-life measured in hours.

Legionella species. It maintains a high degree of activity against β–lactamase-producing *H influenzae* and *M catarrhalis*. It appears to be clinically comparable to cefaclor and amoxicillin/clavulanic acid, and the relatively long half-life allows twice-daily dosing.

■ Cefetamet Pivoxil

Cefetamet pivoxil is an oral third-generation cephalosporin. It is the pivaloyloxymethylester of the semisynthetic third-generation aminothiazolyl cephalosporin, cefetamet. Cefetamet pivoxil has excellent *in vitro* activity against:

- *S pneumoniae*
- *H influenzae*
- *M catarrhalis*
- *Streptococcus pyogenes.*

It is active against β–lactamase-producing strains of *H influenzae* and *M catarrhalis*. It has poor activity against penicillin-resistant *S pneumoniae*, as well as staphylococci and *Pseudomonas* species. The oral bioavailability of cefetamet pivoxil is about 50% after food; drug administration is recommended within 1 hour of a meal. The mean peak plasma concentration of 4 mg/L is attained 4 hours after a single 500-mg dose of cefetamet pivoxil, the plasma elimination half-life is 2.2 to 2.6 hours. Cefetamet is cleared predominantly by the kidneys, and dosage adjustment is needed in patients with renal impairment.

The recommended dosage is 500 mg bid, and in children under 12 years of age, it is 10 mg/kg bid. A dosage of 1000 mg bid is recommended for use against less-sensitive isolates. Cefetamet pivoxil is an effective alternative oral therapy for outpatient treatment of community-acquired respiratory tract infections, especially when there is concern about β-lactamase resistance. Along with all of the cephalosporins, it is not active against the atypical organisms.

■ Cefpodoxime Proxetil

Cefpodoxime proxetil is an orally administered prodrug which is absorbed and de-esterified to release the third-generation cephalosporin cefpodoxime. Cefpodoxime is highly active against both *H influenzae* and *M catarrhalis*, including β–lactamase-producing strains. It is also active against *S pyogenes* and *S pneumoniae,* while penicillin-resistant strains of *S pneumoniae* are moderately susceptible to cefpodoxime. Most strains of *Staphylococcus epidermidis* and *S aureus* are moderately susceptible to cefpodoxime, although the drug is inactive against methicillin-resistant strains of *S aureus*. *P aeruginosa* is resistant to cefpodoxime.

The active metabolite, cefpodoxime, has approximately 50% systemic availability. Bioavailability is significantly increased by food, whereas it is significantly reduced by agents which elevate gastric pH. Peak plasma concentrations of 2.1 to 3.1 mg/L are achieved 2 to 3 hours after single-dose administration of 200 mg, and plasma half-life is 2.1 to 3.6 hours. The drug is eliminated primarily by renal excretion. Cefpodoxime demonstrates a potent inhibitory activity against the common respiratory pathogens (including β–lactamase-producing strains) and has the advantage of moderate activity against penicillin-resistant strains of *S pneumoniae*. It provides effective step-down therapy from parenterally administered third-generation cephalosporins in the treatment of serious respiratory infections.

■ Ceftibuten

Ceftibuten is an orally active third-generation cephalosporin. Ceftibuten has excellent *in vitro* activity against several major respiratory pathogens, including:

- β–Lactamase-positive pathogens

- Negative strains of *H influenzae* and *M catarrhalis*
- *S pyogenes*
- Most strains of Enterobacteriaceae.

Ceftibuten has borderline activity against penicillin-sensitive strains of *S pneumoniae* (MIC_{90} 4 to 8 mg/L). It is inactive against penicillin-resistant strains of *S pneumoniae* and against staphylococci, *Pseudomonas*, enterococci and *Listeria* species. The bioavailability of ceftibuten following oral administration is excellent, ranging between 75% and 90%. Peak plasma concentrations of 10 to 12 mg/L were reached approximately 1.8 hours after administration of ceftibuten 200 mg. The rate and/or extent of absorption of ceftibuten was decreased when administered in doses > 400 mg and when administered with food. The mean elimination half-life of ceftibutin is approximately 2.7 hours in healthy persons and is prolonged to 13.4 hours in patients with severe renal impairment.

Ceftibuten, 400 mg once daily, is the recommended dosage. Despite its rather poor activity against *S pneumoniae*, the results of clinical trials are encouraging. Presumably the excellent pharmacokinetics (high bioavailability, high blood levels, prolonged half-life) compensate for the reduced microbiologic activity.

■ Loracarbef

The carbacephems are a new synthetic class of β-lactam antibiotics which are structurally similar to cephalosporins but with enhanced chemical stability. Loracarbef is the first available drug of this class. *In vitro*, loracarbef shows good activity against:
- *S pneumoniae*
- *S pyogenes*
- *S aureus*
- *M catarrhalis*

- *H influenzae*, including β–lactamase-producing strains.

Like many other β-lactams, an increase in the inoculum size from 10^4 to 10^7 increased the MIC of loracarbef for β–lactamase-resistant strains of bacteria. Methicillin-resistant staphylococci and many Enterobacteriaceae are resistant to loracarbef. After oral administration of a 400-mg capsule, a peak plasma concentration of 12 mg/L is obtained in 1.1 to 1.3 hours and is minimally affected by food. The elimination half-life of loracarbef is 1.1 hours, and excretion is primarily by the renal route.

Adjustment in dosage should be made in moderate to severe renal impairment. For loracarbef, 200 or 400 mg bid is the recommended dosage. It would not be the best choice in severely ill patients or in cases where there is a strong suspicion of gram-negative pathogens.

■ Cefprozil

Cefprozil is an orally active second-generation cephalosporin. Its structure differs from that of other cephalosporins by the addition of a 1-propenyl substituent group at C-3 and a p-hydroxy-phenyl moiety at C-7. The antibacterial spectrum of cefprozil is similar to that of cefaclor, another second-generation cephalosporin. Major respiratory pathogens that are inhibited by cefprozil include:
- *S pyogenes*
- *S pneumoniae*
- *S aureus*
- *H influenzae*
- *M catarrhalis*.

Against β–lactamase-producing strains of *H influenzae* and penicillin-resistant strains of *S pneumoniae,* this drug is generally more active than cefaclor and cephalexin. Enterobacteriaceae are moderately susceptible to cefprozil. Peak plasma concentrations of 5.7 to 18.3 mg/L are obtained within 1 to 2 hours of ingestion and are not significantly affected by food intake. The mean elimination half-life is 1 to 1.4 hours. The majority of the drug is recovered unchanged in the urine, and a dosage reduction is recommended in patients with severe renal dysfunction.

The recommended dosage is 500 mg bid. In three randomized clinical trials of patients with community-acquired lower respiratory tract infections, cefprozil 500 mg bid was as efficacious as cefaclor 500 mg tid, and amoxicillin/clavulanate 500 mg tid, both in clinical response and in bacterial eradication. Cefprozil 500 mg bid, is an effective alternative in the treatment of CAP and is possibly superior to other second-generation cephalosporins in infections caused by β–lactamase-producing organisms.

■ Ceftriaxone

Ceftriaxone is a parenteral third-generation cephalosporin with broad-spectrum *in vitro* activity. *H influenzae* (including β–lactamase-producing strains), *S pneumoniae* (including penicillin-resistant strains) and most Enterobacteriaceae are highly sensitive to the drug. *P aeruginosa* and *Acinetobacter* species are resistant to ceftriaxone. Methicillin-sensitive *S aureus* and *Streptococcus* species are generally susceptible to ceftriaxone, but the drug is not active against methicillin-resistant *S aureus* (MRSA). *S aureus* bacteria should not be treated with ceftriaxone as failures are likely to occur.

Mean peak plasma concentrations are 151 and 257 mg/L following 30-minute infusions of 1 and 2 g intravenously. Trough concentrations are 9.3 and 12 to 20 mg/L (total drug) and 0.5 and 1.2 mg/L (free drug). These are still above the MIC_{90}s of most respiratory pathogens. Adequate concentrations of drug have been measured in most body tissues and fluids, including purulent sputum, bronchial mucosa and lung tissue. Approximately two thirds of a dose are eliminated via glomerular filtration, while the rest is excreted mainly in the bile. Dosage adjustments in the presence of moderate renal or hepatic disease are not necessary.

Many clinical trials have established the efficacy of this agent in CAP and HAP. Third-generation cephalosporins, such as ceftriaxone, are generally recommended as initial empiric therapy for serious infections such as nosocomial pneumonia or severe CAP. However, ceftriaxone, like most other third-generation cephalosporins, should not be administered empirically in patients with severe HAP of unknown etiology if *P aeruginosa* is the suspected pathogen.

■ Ceftazidime

Ceftazidime is an aminothiazolyl, third-generation cephalosporin, antibacterial agent whose action is mediated, like other agents in this class, through binding with PBPs and inhibiting the cross-linking of bacterial peptidoglycan. *In vitro* data from many countries suggest that in general, the common nosocomial pathogens of Enterobacteriaceae such as *E coli, K pneumoniae* and *Proteus mirabilis* remain highly susceptible to ceftazidime. Activity against other important gram-negative pathogens such as *Enterobacter* species and *Serratia marcescens* is less predictable and may encourage the emergence of extended spectrum β–lactamase-producing organisms. There is a wide range of susceptibility of *P aeruginosa,* with approximately 85% of strains remaining susceptible. Ceftazidime remains active against the respiratory tract pathogens *H influenzae* and *M catarrhalis.* However, it is not active against MRSA, and ceftazidime is less active than the other parenteral agents against penicillin-resistant pneumococci.

Following the administration of a 1- and 2-g intravenous dose, a maximum serum concentration (C_{max}) of 59 to 83 mg/L and 159 to 185 mg/L, respectively, can be anticipated. Ceftazidime is renally excreted, and dosage adjustments are required with renal insufficiency. Adequate concentrations have been reported in bronchial secretions, lung tissue and pleural fluid. Ceftazidime, either as monotherapy or as a component of an antibacterial regimen, remains effective in the treatment of serious nosocomial infections, especially those associated with gram-negative bacteria. The usual adult dosage is 3 to 6 g/d by intravenous infusion or injection given tid. Higher doses may be required in patients with cystic fibrosis, and dosage reduction is essential in patients with renal impairment.

■ Cefepime

Cefepime is a fourth-generation parenteral cephalosporin with activity against both gram-positive and gram-negative aerobic bacteria. Cefepime has greater inhibitory activity than ceftazidime against *S pneumoniae* and staphylococcal species. Similar to other cephalosporins, it is not active against MRSA. A useful feature of this agent, in contrast to previous generations of cephalosporins, is that it maintains its activity against depressed bacteria. In addition, cefepime is not susceptible to hydrolysis by plasmid-mediated β-lactamases expressed by gram-negative bacteria, particularly *Enterobacter* species. Unlike imipenem and some second-generation cephalosporins, cefepime is a poor inducer of type I β-lactamases. Cefepime has activity similar to that of ceftazidime against *P aeruginosa*.

A dose of 2 g intravenously will produce a C_{max} of 126 to 193 mg/L. It has an elimination half-life of approximately 2 hours, allowing twice daily dosing. Plasma protein binding is low, and the drug distributes widely into body tissues and fluids. Renal clearance of the drug dictates a reduction in dosage in the presence of significant renal insufficiency. Cefepime, administered 2 g bid, is comparable in clinical and microbiologic efficacy to ceftazidime administered 2 g tid or cefotaxime 2 g tid in patients with nosocomial and community-acquired lower respiratory tract infections.

■ Imipenem/Cilastatin

Imipenem is the N-formimidoyl derivative of thienamycin, a β-lactam antibiotic produced by *Streptomyces cattleya*. It is coadministered with cilastatin, a specific inhibitor of the renal enzyme dehydropeptidase-1 (DHP-1), to prevent rapid renal metabolism of imipenem. Imipenem is active against a wide range of Enterobacteriaceae, including a greater proportion of *Enterobacter cloacae* and *Citrobacter freundii* than third- or fourth-generation cephalosporins. It is generally less active than ciprofloxacin against *E coli*, *K pneumoniae*, *E cloacae* and *S marcescens*. Imipenem has excellent activity against methicillin-susceptible *S aureus*, *S pyogenes* and *S pneumoniae*. The activity against the *Bacteroides fragilis* group, other *Bacteroides* and *Clostridium* species is comparable to that of metronidazole. Although a strong inducer of class I β-lactamases, imipenem is not hydrolyzed by these enzymes and has remained active against a wide range of β–lactamase- and non–β-lactamase-producing bacteria.

Single-dose intravenous administration of imipenem/cilastatin 500 mg or 1000 mg results in mean plasma concentrations of 30 to 35 mg/L and 60 to 70 mg/L, respectively, which decline to 0.5 and 2 mg/L, respectively, 4 to 6 hours later. The elimination half-life of both imipenem and cilastatin is about 1 hour after intravenous administration. In patients with severely impaired renal function, the elimination half-life of cilastatin is prolonged to a greater degree than that of imipenem. In severe lower respiratory tract infections, addition of an aminoglycoside has been recommended to reduce the likelihood of development of resistant *P aeruginosa*. Seizures have occurred in patients with central nervous system dysfunction and renal failure, in conjunction with unadjusted dosage regimens. The usual intravenous dose is 500 to 750 mg administered every 6 hours, depending on the severity of the infection.

■ **Meropenem**

Meropenem is a broad-spectrum carbapenem antibacterial agent that is stable in the presence of DHP-1 such that it does not require concomitant administration of a DHP-1 inhibitor such as cilastatin. The drug is generally more active than imipenem against Enterobacteriaceae, including nosocomial clinical isolates resistant to ceftazidime, cefotaxime, ceftriaxone, piperacillin and gentamicin. Meropenem is active against *S aureus* but is less active than imipenem against other gram-positive organisms. *S pneumoniae*, including penicillin-resistant strains, is inhibited by low concentrations of meropenem. It is as active or more active than imipenem against anaerobic bacteria.

After a 30-minute intravenous infusion of 1 g of meropenem, the peak plasma concentration varies from 53 to 61 mg/L. The elimination half-life is approximately 1 hour, and the excretion is mainly renal. Randomized trials indicate clinical efficacy in patients with lower respiratory tract infections similar to that with imipenem/cilastatin and ceftazidime, with or without an aminoglycoside. The recommended intravenous dosage of meropenem is 0.5 to 1 g every 8 hours, which should be decreased in the presence of renal insufficiency.

Macrolides

Until recently, erythromycin has been the principal compound in the class of macrolides. These drugs have been used extensively in the treatment of lower respiratory tract infections, especially in patients allergic to β-lactam antibiotics or with infections due to intracellular organisms (*Chlamydia*, *Legionella* and *Toxoplasma* species) and atypical pathogens such as *Mycoplasma* species. The activity of erythromycin against gram-negative species is poor. Macrolide antibiotics exhibit their antimicrobial action by binding to the 50S subunit of the 70S ribosome, thereby inhibiting bacterial RNA-dependent protein synthesis. Erythromycin has poor oral bioavailability requiring dosing 3 to 4 times a day, is unstable in an acid environment and lacks efficacy against *H influenzae*. Although not serious, the drug causes dose-related GI symptoms, including nausea, vomiting and diarrhea. The intravenous formulation of the drug causes severe local phlebitis and requires a large volume for administration.

Its 14-membered ring has now been modified to produce semisynthetic derivatives, including clarithromycin, roxithromycin, dirithromycin and others. Azithromycin is a 15-membered ring, which confers upon it acid stability. These new compounds have an increased spectrum of activity, demonstrate increased stability in acid solutions and are better tolerated following oral administration. MIC_{90} values are summarized in Table 5.4 and pharmacokinetic properties are compared in Table 5.5. Common drug interactions are listed in Table 5.6.

■ Clarithromycin

Clarithromycin is a 14-membered lactone ring attached to two sugar moieties. The primary metabolite of clarithromycin is the 14-hydroxy(R) epimer,

TABLE 5.4 — *IN VITRO* MIC$_{90}$ VALUES (MG/L) OF MACROLIDES AGAINST SELECTED RESPIRATORY PATHOGENS

Organism	Azithromycin	Clarithromycin	Dirithromycin	Erythromycin	Roxithromycin
Chlamydia pneumoniae	0.06-4	0.007-0.015	—	0.06	0.06-4
Haemophilus influenzae	0.25-1	2-8*	8- > 16	2-8	4-16
Legionella species	2	0.025	16	2	0.5
Moraxella catarrhalis	0.06	0.12-0.25	0.25	0.25	0.5-1
Streptococcus pneumoniae	0.015-0.25	0.015-0.06	0.06-0.12	0.015-0.25	0.03-0.12
Streptococcus pyogenes	0.03-4	0.015-0.25	0.12-2	0.03-4	0.06-2

Abbreviations: MIC$_{90}$, minimum inhibitory concentration inhibiting 90% of tested strains.

* MIC$_{90}$ or clarithromycin alone. With 14-OH metabolite, MIC$_{90}$ may be lower.

TABLE 5.5 — PHARMACOKINETIC PROPERTIES OF MACROLIDES

Drug	Dose (mg)	T_{max} (h)	Tissue Concentration* (mg/kg)	C_{max} (mg/L)	$t\frac{1}{2} B$ (h)
Azithromycin	500 od	2.5-2.6	4.74†	0.62	10-40
Clarithromycin	500 bid	2.2-2.3	17.47	2.4-3.5	3.3-3.5
Dirithromycin	500 od	4-4.5	3.8	0.48	42
Erythromycin	500 bid	1.9-4.4	4.2	3	2
Roxithromycin	150 bid	2.4	5.64	6.8	13

Abbreviations: T_{max}, time to maximum serum concentration; C_{max}, maximum serum concentration; $t\frac{1}{2} B$, terminal half-life measured in hours.

* Lung tissue unless otherwise stated.
† Bronchial mucosa.

TABLE 5.6 — COMMON DRUG INTERACTIONS WITH THE MACROLIDES
Azithromycin   • Reduced absorption with antacids   • Increased effect of warfarin sodium (Coumadin)   • Increased theophylline levels
Clarithromycin   • Elevates theophylline levels   • Cisapride-induced ventricular arrhythmias   • Increased carbamazepine levels
Erythromycin   • Increased theophylline levels   • Increased digoxin levels   • Increased effect of warfarin sodium (Coumadin)   • Increased cyclosporine toxicity   • Cisapride-induced ventricular arrhythmias

which also has antimicrobial activity, and this has been shown to be additive or synergistic to that of the parent compound against a variety of bacteria, particularly *H influenzae*. Clarithromycin has a spectrum of antimicrobial activity similar to that of erythromycin with activity against:

- *S pneumoniae*
- *S aureus*
- β-Hemolytic *Streptococcus*
- *S pyogenes*
- *M pneumoniae*
- *M catarrhalis* (including β–lactamase-producing strains).

Bacterial strains resistant to erythromycin are also resistant to clarithromycin. However, clarithromycin demonstrates greater *in vitro* activity than erythromycin against certain respiratory pathogens, including *C pneumoniae*, *Legionella* species and *H influenzae*. It also exhibits a potent postantibiotic effect against *S aureus*, *S pneumoniae* and *H influenzae*.

Clarithromycin is well absorbed from the GI tract, but undergoes substantial first-pass metabolism, reducing systemic bioavailability to 55%. Macrolides are lipid-soluble, resulting in extensive body fluid and tissue distribution. In animal and human studies, clarithromycin has achieved greater concentrations in tissues and organs than in blood. The mean elimination half-life ranges from 2.6 to 2.8 hours, while the half-life for the 14-hydroxy(R) epimer is greater than that of the parent compound (3.9 to 5.1 hours) after single-dose administration. The recommended oral dosage of clarithromycin for the treatment of pneumonia is 250 or 500 mg bid taken with or without food.

The clinical success rate for clarithromycin in patients with lower respiratory tract infections is 94% to 99%. In summary, clarithromycin is effective against most respiratory tract pathogens causing pneumonia, including atypical pathogens (eg, *C pneumoniae*, *M pneumoniae*, and *Legionella* species). Use of this agent may be preferred in patients with underlying lung disease who are at an increased risk of infections caused by β–lactamase-producing organisms such as *H influenzae* and *M catarrhalis*. Its pharmacokinetic properties are superior to those of erythromycin, allowing twice-daily dosing with the potential for greater compliance.

■ **Azithromycin**

Azithromycin is a 15-membered ring erythromycin analogue with a nitrogen inserted into the lactone ring; this confers acid stability and improved tissue pharmacokinetic properties. Azithromycin is the prototype of the semisynthetic macrolides known as the azalides. Azithromycin is marginally less active than erythromycin *in vitro* against gram-positive organisms and has similar activity against atypical intracellular pathogens (eg, *C pneumoniae, L pneumophila, M pneumoniae*). It is more active than other new macrolides against many gram-negative pathogens, including *H influenzae, Haemophilus parainfluenzae* and *M catarrhalis*. Like other macrolides, it is unaffected by β-lactamase production. However, erythromycin-resistant strains are generally azithromycin- and clarithromycin-resistant as well.

Following oral administration, azithromycin is rapidly cleared from the circulation into intracellular compartments, resulting in high tissue concentrations. The oral bioavailability of a single 500-mg dose in a fasting state is 37%. It is then released slowly, demonstrating a long terminal elimination half-life (10 to 40 hours) compared with that of erythromycin (1.7 hours). Azithromycin is eliminated unchanged principally in the feces and to a lesser extent via the kidneys. Azithromycin is usually given as a single or divided 500-mg dose on day 1 followed by 250 mg once daily for an additional 4 days. Azithromycin should be given at least 1 hour before or 2 hours after food or antacids. It is recommended that azithromycin be used with caution in patients with severe renal impairment and not used at all in those with severe hepatic disease.

In comparative studies, azithromycin shows overall efficacy comparable with that of erythromycin, josamycin, amoxicillin (with or without clavulanic acid) or cefaclor. Azithromycin is an orally active, acid-stable antimicrobial that offers an effective alternative to erythromycin in the treatment of lower respiratory tract infections. It has the best gram-negative coverage of all the available macrolides but does not cover *Enterobacter* or *Pseudomonas* species. The possibility of once-daily administration and a shorter duration of treatment due to its pharmacokinetic properties is attractive as a means of improving patient compliance and possibly lowering overall costs of treatment.

■ Roxithromycin

Roxithromycin is a semisynthetic derivative of erythromycin modified at the C-9 position. The *in vitro* activity of roxithromycin resembles that of the parent compound. It is active against:

- *S pneumoniae*
- *S pyogenes*
- *M catarrhalis*
- *L pneumophila*
- *M pneumoniae*
- *Chlamydia trachomatis.*

Activity against *H influenzae* is borderline. It has variable activity against methicillin-susceptible *S aureus*. Bioavailability is reduced when the drug is administered 15 minutes after a standard meal; therefore, it is recommended that it be given at least 15 minutes before food. The mean elimination half-life of roxithromycin (8.4 to 15.5 hours) is much longer than that of the parent compound, erythromycin (1.5 to 3 hours). The drug is strongly and saturably bound to alpha-1-acid glycoprotein in plasma from which it is released for distribution and elimination. This may be the mechanism for its nonlinear pharmacokinetics. Roxithromycin is primarily excreted in the feces. A 50% reduction in daily dose has been recommended in patients with liver cirrhosis.

The recommended daily oral dosage of roxithromycin in adults is 300 mg administered either once daily or in two divided doses. A reduced dose of 150 mg is recommended in patients with liver cirrhosis, but no dosage adjustment is required in severe renal failure. In summary, it should not be used in cases where infection due to *H influenzae* is likely. It is useful in people with severe renal failure since most of its elimination is hepatic. The long elimination half-life allows for once or twice daily dosing, and it is better tolerated than erythromycin.

■ Dirithromycin

Dirithromycin is an orally active macrolide with a 14-membered lactone ring. It is readily hydrolyzed to its biologically active metabolite, erythromycylamine. The *in vitro* inhibitory activity of dirithromycin against gram-positive clinical isolates is similar to that of the other macrolides, erythromycin, roxithromycin and azithromycin, and generally less than that of clarithromycin. The spectrum of activity includes:

- *S pneumoniae*
- *S pyogenes*
- Penicillin-sensitive strains of *S aureus*
- *Listeria monocytogenes*
- *M catarrhalis* (including some β–lactamase-producing strains)
- Atypical pathogens.

Dirithromycin has no relevant activity against *Brucella* species, and some strains of *H influenzae*. Its activity against *L pneumophila* is inferior to that of other macrolide antibiotics. Dirithromycin is rapidly converted by nonenzymatic hydrolysis to the active metabolite, erythromycylamine. Systemic availability is 10%, and food has a minimal effect on absorption. The drug rapidly leaves the circulation and localizes in selected soft tissues and has a long elimination half-life of 28 (16 to 60) hours. Elimination is primarily by liver and feces.

The suggested dosage of dirithromycin is 500 mg once daily in adults. No dosage reduction is required in patients with mild to moderate hepatic or renal impairment. Dirithromycin is similar to erythromycin in its microbiologic spectrum of activity as well as in its tolerability. The high tissue penetration, slow efflux from tissues and cells and longer half-life result in a more convenient once-daily dosing. Further comparative studies with the other new members of the macrolide class are required.

Fluoroquinolones

Fluoroquinolones exert their effect by inhibiting DNA gyrase, thereby inhibiting DNA synthesis. In general, the fluoroquinolones have excellent activity against gram-negative pulmonary pathogens such as:

- *H influenzae*
- Enterobacteriaceae
- *Pseudomonas* species (ciprofloxacin only).

Streptococci are less susceptible and activity against anaerobes is poor, especially in the earlier versions of fluoroquinolones. Atypical pathogens such as *M pneumoniae* and *Chlamydia* species are variably susceptible, and *Legionella* species are inhibited by fluoroquinolones. MIC_{90} values are displayed in Table 5.7. The fluoroquinolones and their dosing are shown in Table 5.8, while the concentration of the fluoroquinolones in lung tissue is demonstrated in Table 5.9. The relationship between the pharmacokinetics, pharmacodynamics and MIC_{90} values of the newer fluoroquinolones against *S pneumoniae* is shown in Table 5.10. Since bacterial killing of fluoroquinolones is concentration-dependent, a fluoroquinolone with a concentration significantly above the MIC_{90} (as reflected by a high area under the curve above the concentration required to inhibit 90% of strains [AUIC]) would be expected to be successful in eradicating this pathogen.

TABLE 5.7 — *IN VITRO* MIC$_{90}$ VALUES (MG/L) OF ORAL FLUOROQUINOLONES AGAINST SELECTED RESPIRATORY PATHOGENS

Organism	Cipro	Grepa	Levo	Moxi	Spar	Trova
Haemophilus influenzae	0.02	0.008	0.02	0.06	0.05	0.05
Klebsiella pneumoniae	0.06	0.25	0.5	0.13	0.12	0.12
Moraxella catarrhalis	0.01-0.25	0.004-0.03	0.09	0.004-0.03	0.01-0.12	0.002-0.03
Pseudomonas aeruginosa	4	8	8	8	8	8
Staphylococcus aureus	0.5-0.78	—	0.41	0.06	0.1	0.39
Streptococcus pneumoniae	2	0.5	1.91	0.12	0.5	0.12
Streptococcus pyogenes	0.78	—	1.26	0.25	1.56	0.78

Abbreviations: MIC$_{90}$, minimum inhibitory concentration inhibiting 90% of strains; Cipro, ciprofloxacin; Grepa, grepafloxacin; Levo, levofloxacin; Moxi, moxifloxacin; Spar, sparfloxacin; Trova, trovafloxacin.

TABLE 5.8 — FLUOROQUINOLONES USED IN COMMUNITY-ACQUIRED PNEUMONIA		
Drug	**Spectrum of Activity**	**Dose**
Ciprofloxacin	*Pseudomonas aeruginosa*, gram-negatives	750 mg po/bid/d
Grepafloxacin	*Pneumococcus, Mycoplasma, Chlamydia, Legionella*	400-600 mg po/d
Levofloxacin	Gram-negatives, *Pneumococcus, Mycoplasma, Chlamydia, Legionella*	500 mg po/d
Moxifloxacin	*Pneumococcus*, gram-negatives, *Mycoplasma, Chlamydia, Legionella*	400 mg po/d
Sparfloxacin	*Pneumococcus, Mycoplasma, Chlamydia, Legionella* species	400 mg po 1st dose then 200 mg po qd

TABLE 5.9 — ACCUMULATION OF QUINOLONES IN LUNG TISSUES

Fluoroquinolone	Oral Dose (mg)	C_{max} (mg/L)	Bronchial Mucosa (mg/L)	Epithelial Lining Fluid (mg/L)	Alveolar Macrophage (mg/L)
Ciprofloxacin	250 bid × 4 d	1.1	1.8	2.0	14.8
Grepafloxacin	600	1.8	5.3	27.1	27.6
Levofloxacin	500	6.6	8.3	10.9	41.9
Moxifloxacin	400	3.3	5.5	24.4	113.6
Sparfloxacin	400	0.5	1.3	5.6	9.6
Trovafloxacin	200	1.4	1.5	4.0	19.1

Abbreviation: C_{max}, maximum serum concentration.

TABLE 5.10 — ACTIVITY OF FLUOROQUINOLONES AGAINST *STREPTOCOCCUS PNEUMONIAE*							
Fluoroquinolone	Dose (mg)	C_{max} (mg/L)	AUC (mg/L·h)	MIC_{90} (mg/L)	C_{max}:MIC_{90}	AUIC (mg/L·h)	Protein Binding (%)
Grepafloxacin	400	1.4	11.0	0.25	5.6	44	50
Levofloxacin	500	5.7	47.5	1-2	3-6	24-48	24-38
Moxifloxacin	400	4.5	48.0	0.12-0.25	18-37.5	192-400	30-45
Sparfloxacin	200	1.4	32.7	0.5	3	65	45
Trovafloxacin	200	3.1	3.4	0.12-0.5	12.4-26	138-287	70-88

Abbreviations: C_{max}, maximum serum concentration; AUC, area under the concentration time curve; MIC_{90}, minimum inhibitory concentration inhibiting 90% of strains; AUIC, area under the curve above the concentration required to inhibit 90% of strains.

■ Ciprofloxacin

Ciprofloxacin is the benchmark fluoroquinolone against which all other fluoroquinolones are compared (Table 5.8). It is the only fluoroquinolone available in oral, IV, otic and optic formulations. The primary mechanism of action is inhibition of bacterial DNA gyrase, which disrupts bacterial DNA replication. Ciprofloxacin is active *in vitro* against most gram-negative bacteria, including *M catarrhalis* and *H influenzae*. *S pneumoniae*, including penicillin-resistant strains, is generally susceptible or moderately susceptible (MIC$_{90}$ 1 or 2 mg/L).

Ciprofloxacin has a bioavailabilty of approximately 70% after oral administration and reaches a C$_{max}$ of 3.9 mg/L 1 to 2 hours after a single 750-mg dose. It is concentrated in many body tissues and fluids, particularly lung tissue and alveolar macrophages. Clearance is mainly renal and age-related adjustments in dosage may be necessary. Despite the concern regarding the marginal *S pneumoniae* activity, the clinical and bacteriologic efficacy of ciprofloxacin is similar to that of more traditional agents. It has been used successfully in the management of chronic obstructive pulmonary disease exacerbations and acute bronchitis where *S pneumoniae* is a prominent pathogen. However, its use in primary pneumococcal pneumonia is not encouraged.

■ Levofloxacin

Levofloxacin is an oral and intravenous fluoroquinolone which is the optical S-(-)isomer of ofloxacin. Its *in vitro* activity is generally twice as potent as that of ofloxacin. Levofloxacin demonstrates better gram-positive coverage than previous fluoroquinolones against both methicillin-sensitive and methicillin-resistant *S aureus* and most *Streptococcus* species. Ciprofloxacin is twice as potent as levofloxacin against many gram-negative bacteria and is more active against *P aeruginosa*. The oral bioavailability of levofloxacin is close to 100% and is unaffected by food. Maximum plasma drug concentrations of 1.1 to 1.3 mg/L are reached in 0.8 to 2.4 hours. Concentrations of drug in tissues or body fluids are generally higher than those observed in plasma, due to the wide distribution of the drug throughout the body. The mean plasma elimination half-life is 4 to 7 hours. Excretion occurs primarily through the urine, and dosage adjustment is necessary in patients with impaired renal function.

The usual dose is 500 mg once daily. This should **5** not be administered to children or pregnant or lactating women due to the potential for articular damage. Patients should not receive concomitant mineral supplements, vitamins, iron or other minerals, antacids or sucralfate. Levofloxacin possesses comparable or better activity than ciprofloxacin and ofloxacin against gram-positive bacteria which are pathogens in pneumonia. It should not be used where infection due to *P aeruginosa* is strongly suspected.

■ **Trovafloxacin**

Trovafloxacin is a new fluoronaphthyridone recently released in oral and intravenous formulations. It is structurally distinct from previous fluoroquinolones. Trovafloxacin has gram-positive coverage that is superior to that of previous fluoroquinolones. It has potent activity against MRSA, coagulase-negative staphylococcci, *S pyogenes* and penicillin-resistant *S pneumoniae*. It is also active against gram-negative respiratory pathogens such as *H influenzae*, *C pneumoniae*, *M catarrhalis*, and *Legionella* species. Anaerobes have been found to be highly susceptible to this compound.

Trovafloxacin is rapidly absorbed after oral administration and peak plasma concentrations are reached in 0.7 to 3.3 hours. The overall half-life is

10.5 hours. It is 70% bound to serum proteins. Less than 10% of the dose is excreted in urine, most of the excretion is through the biliary route. The pharmacokinetics allows for once-daily administration. The dose for respiratory tract infections is in the range of 100 to 300 mg. Trovafloxacin is the first fluoroquinolone to offer improved gram-positive and anaerobic coverage. Its long half-life and excellent oral absorption will allow a more convenient dosing schedule.

Unfortunately, liver toxicity has been identified with the use of this drug. Initially, the toxicity was associated with prolonged administration of the drug, but more recent experience has demonstrated that liver toxicity is unpredictable and the drug essentially has been withdrawn from community practice. The drug will remain available for parenteral usage in a hospital setting.

■ Grepafloxacin

Grepafloxacin is a new oral monofluorinated fluoroquinolone with a novel methyl substitute at position 7. It has high tissue penetration and a wide spectrum of activity, with improved activity against *S pneumoniae*. Grepafloxacin is 8 to 16 times more active than ofloxacin against *Chlamydia* species and fourfold more active against *M pneumoniae*. It has an MIC against *Legionella* species ranging from 0.008 to 0.03 mg/L, equivalent to that seen with ofloxacin, clarithromycin and rifampin. It is rapidly absorbed and reaches peak concentration after 2 hours. It has an extended half-life of approximately 12 hours. Grepafloxacin is eliminated primarily through metabolism and is excreted in feces. Renal impairment does not affect grepafloxacin pharmacokinetics, whereas peak plasma concentrations, areas under the plasma concentration-time curves (AUCs) and renal excretion are increased in patients with hepatic impairment.

Lung concentrations are among the highest seen with any of the fluoroquinolones. Theophylline clearance is approximately halved during coadministration with grepafloxacin, and therefore the maintenance dose of theophylline should be halved if the two drugs are to be given simultaneously. No dosage adjustment is warranted if warfarin and grepafloxacin are given concurrently. The usual dose recommended for the treatment of pneumonia is 600 mg given once daily.

■ Sparfloxacin

Sparfloxacin is a new fluoroquinolone, chemically related to other new fluoroquinolones. Its antimicrobial activity is similar to that of many of the other newer fluoroquinolones. It is active against most gram-negative rods, with *P aeruginosa* being the major exception. It is also active against non–methicillin-resistant *S aureus* as well as *S pneumoniae* but lacks activity against *Bacteroides fragilis* and other anaerobic organisms. It has excellent activity against *M pneumoniae*, *C pneumoniae* and *L pneumophila*.

After a 400-mg dose, peak serum levels are generally 3.0 mg/mL with a prolonged elimination half-life. Sparfloxacin can be used for the treatment of CAP. It has a higher incidence of photosensitivity reactions than many of the other newer fluoroquinolones, thus limiting its use, and patients must be cautioned to avoid the sun when taking this medication. The usual dosage is 400 mg taken on the first day as a loading dose, and then 200 mg qd for 10 days.

■ Moxifloxacin

Moxifloxcin is a new 8-methoxyquinolone with a broad spectrum of activity. It covers all of the usual respiratory pathogens, including the atypical organisms, while maintaining an excellent gram-negative spectrum. A single dose of 400 mg produces a C_{max} of 3.2 to 4.5 mg/L, half-life of 11 to 15 hours, AUC of 25 to 40 mg/L per hour and volume of distribution of 2.5 to 3.5 L/kg. Bioavailability is > 85% and elimination is by metabolic, renal and biliary/fecal pathways. Approximately 20% of the clearance is via the kidneys. The drug concentrates in bronchial mucosa, lung epithelial fluid and alveolar macrophages at concentrations that are considerably higher than that required to kill the common respiratory pathogens. The concentrations seen in the lung with this drug are the highest identified of the available or soon to be released fluoroquinolones. No dosage adjustment is required with renal failure and there are no important drug interactions except with antacids and iron or other divalent cation preparations similar to all the other fluoroquinolones. Clinical trials have demonstrated bacteriological and/or clinical success rates of approximately 90% or greater for CAP, acute exacerbation of chronic bronchitis or acute sinusitis. It is the only fluoroquinolone that has received regulatory authority approval for use against penicillin-non–susceptible strains of *S pneumoniae*. The usual dosage is 400 mg taken once daily.

SUGGESTED READING

Bahal N, Nahata MC. The new macrolide antibiotics: azithromycin, clarithromycin, dirithromycin, and roxithromycin. *Ann Pharmacother*. 1992;26:46-55.

Barradell LB, Bryson HM. Cefepime. A review of its antibacterial activity, pharmacokinetic properties and therapeutic use. *Drugs*. 1994;47:471-505.

Brogden RN, McTavish D. Loracarbef. A review of its antimicrobial activity, pharmacokinetic properties and therapeutic efficacy. *Drugs*. 1993;45:716-736.

Brogden RN, Peters DH. Dirithromycin. A review of its antimicrobial activity, pharmacokinetic properties and therapeutic efficacy. *Drugs*. 1994;48:599-616.

Bryson HM, Brogden RN. Cefetamet pivoxil. A review of its antibacterial activity, pharmacokinetic properties and therapeutic use. *Drugs*. 1993;45:589-621.

Buckley MM, Brogden RN, Barradell LB, Goa KL. Imipenem/cilastatin. A reappraisal of its antibacterial activity, pharmacokinetic properties and therapeutic efficacy [published erratum appears in *Drugs*. 1992;44:1012]. *Drugs*. 1992;44:408-444.

Davies AJ, Jolley A. Antibacterial therapy of community-acquired chest infections. *J Antimicrob Chemother*. 1992;29:1-4.

Davis R, Bryson HM. Levofloxacin. A review of its antibacterial activity, pharmacokinetics and therapeutic efficacy [published erratum appears in *Drugs*. 1994;48:132]. *Drugs*. 1994;47:677-700.

Davis R, Markham A, Balfour JA. Ciprofloxacin. An updated review of its pharmacology, therapeutic efficacy and tolerability. *Drugs*. 1996;51:1019-1074.

Doern GV. Trends in antimicrobial susceptibility of bacterial pathogens of the respiratory tract. *Am J Med*. 1995;99(suppl 6B):3S-7S.

Foulds G, Shepard RM, Johnson RB. The pharmacokinetics of azithromycin in human serum and tissues. *J Antimicrob Chemother*. 1990;25(suppl A):73-82.

Frampton JE, Brogden RN, Langtry HD, Buckley MM. Cefpodoxime proxetil. A review of its antibacterial activity, pharmacokinetic properties and therapeutic potential. *Drugs*. 1992;44:889-917.

Hooper DC. Quinolone mode of action. *Drugs*. 1995;49(suppl 2):10-15.

Jorgensen JH. Update on mechanisms and prevalence of antimicrobial resistance in *Haemophilus influenzae*. *Clin Infect Dis*. 1992;14:1119-1123.

Kayser FH, Morenzoni G, Santanam P. The Second European Collaborative Study on the frequency of antimicrobial resistance in *Haemophilus influenzae*. *Eur J Clin Microbiol Infect Dis*. 1990; 9:810-817.

Markham A, Faulds D. Roxithromycin. An update of its antimicrobial activity, pharmacokinetic properties and therapeutic use [published erratum appears in *Drugs*. 1994;48:793]. *Drugs*. 1994; 48:297-326.

5

Moellering RC Jr. β-Lactamase inhibition: therapeutic implications in infectious diseases—an overview. *Rev Infect Dis.* 1991;13(suppl 9):S723-S726.

Nilsen OG. Comparative pharmacokinetics of macrolides [published erratum appears in *J Antimicrob Chemother.* 1988;21:813]. *J Antimicrob Chemother.* 1987;20(suppl B):81-88.

Peters DH, Clissold SP. Clarithromycin. A review of its antimicrobial activity, pharmacokinetic properties and therapeutic potential. *Drugs.* 1992;44:117-164.

Peters DH, Friedel HA, McTavish D. Azithromycin. A review of its antimicrobial activity, pharmacokinetic properties and clinical efficacy. *Drugs.* 1992;44:750-799.

Peters G, Pulverer G, Neugebauer M. *In vitro*-activity of clavulanic acid and amoxicillin combined against amoxicillin-resistant bacteria. *Infection.* 1980;8:104-106.

Puri SK, Lassman HB. Roxithromycin: a pharmacokinetic review of a macrolide. *J Antimicrob Chemother.* 1987;20(suppl B):89-100.

Rains CP, Bryson HM, Peters DH. Ceftazidime. An update of its antibacterial activity, pharmacokinetic properties and therapeutic efficacy. *Drugs.* 1995;49:577-617.

Sides GD, Cerimele BJ, Black HR, et al. Pharmacokinetics of dirithromycin. *J Antimicrob Chemother.* 1993;31(suppl C):65-75.

Wise R. A review of the clinical pharmacology of moxifloxacin, a new 8-methoxyquinolone, and its potential relation to therapeutic efficacy. *Clin Drug Invest.* 1999;17:365-387.

Wiseman LR, Balfour JA. Ceftibuten. A review of its antibacterial activity, pharmacokinetic properties and clinical efficacy. *Drugs.* 1994;47:784-808.

Wiseman LR, Benfield P. Cefprozil. A review of its antibacterial activity, pharmacokinetic properties, and therapeutic potential. *Drugs.* 1993;45:295-317.

Wiseman LR, Wagstaff AJ, Brogden RN, Bryson HM. Meropenem. A review of its antibacterial activity, pharmacokinetic properties and clinical efficacy. *Drugs.* 1995;50:73-101.

6 Nosocomial or Hospital-Acquired Pneumonia

Epidemiology

Hospital-acquired pneumonia (HAP) is defined as pneumonia occurring 48 hours after admission to the hospital and excluding those incubating at the time of admission. Patients with tracheal intubation and/or requiring mechanical ventilation have a 6- to 20-fold increased risk for nosocomial pneumonia. There is a relatively constant 1% to 3% risk per day for developing ventilator-associated pneumonia (VAP) in medical and surgical intensive-care units (ICUs). The rates are much lower in nonintubated patients and in those in pediatric ICUs, but higher in adult medical and surgical ICUs and burn units. When compared to matched controls, patients developing VAP have a 2- to 2.5-fold increased risk of mortality.

Crude mortality rates for this disease range from 20% to 71%, but deaths are often due to other causes in critically ill patients. A preferred measure is "attributable mortality" defined as the percentage of deaths that would not have occurred in the absence of the infection. Using matched cohort studies, an attributable mortality of 27% to 33% has been reported. The major risk factors for mortality include:

- Severity of underlying illness
- Inappropriate antibiotic therapy
- Infection with high-risk pathogens such as *Pseudomonas aeruginosa*
- Advanced age.

Rates of secondary bacteremia range from 4% to 38% with a median of 11%. Empyema has been reported following the development of nosocomial pneumonia. Each episode of HAP will prolong a hospital stay by an average of 7 to 9 days, resulting in increased hospital charges. A recent study indicated that costs would exceed reimbursement in the vast majority of Medicare patients developing nosocomial pneumonia.

Risk Factors and Pathogenesis

The respiratory tract is uniquely designed to prevent entry of pathogenic organisms into the lung and to eradicate these microorganisms if they manage to bypass upper airway host defenses. Included in this defense armamentarium are:

- Filtration and humidification of the upper airway
- Cough reflexes
- Mucociliary escalator, an elaborate system that transports secretions and microorganisms from the periphery of the lung to the central airways where they are expectorated or swallowed.

Organisms impact onto the mucous layer because of inertial forces whenever there is a major airway division. Being trapped in this layer, the organisms are removed when oscillating cilia transport the mucus to the central airways. If the organisms reach the periphery of the lung, phagocytes and opsonins remove many of them and systemic humoral and cell-mediated immunity deals with the rest. Pneumonia occurs only when this elaborate defense mechanism is overwhelmed, either because of a large aspirated inoculum or the inherent virulence of organisms, or when the defense mechanism is breached in some manner.

The most common means of acquiring pneumonia is via aspiration of oropharyngeal content. As many as 45% of healthy subjects aspirate during sleep. Aspiration is more likely among patients with:

- Abnormal swallowing
- Impaired gag reflex
- Altered consciousness
- Delayed gastric emptying
- Decreased gastric motility.

Nasogastric tubes may contribute to increased oropharyngeal colonization, either by providing a conduit for organisms to migrate from the stomach or by causing erosions on mucosal surfaces, thereby exposing more binding sites to gram-negative bacilli. A crucial first step in the development of nosocomial pneumonia is the adherence of potential pathogenic organisms to buccal mucosa (Table 6.1). This is facilitated by critical illness when increased levels of salivary proteases degrade cell-surface fibronectin.

Many patients have upper airway colonization with pathogenic bacteria, and the leading organisms associated with nosocomial pneumonia are enteric

TABLE 6.1 — FACTORS ASSOCIATED WITH INCREASED MORTALITY IN NOSOCOMIAL PNEUMONIA

- Aerobic gram-negative pathogens, especially *Pseudomonas aeruginosa*
- Severity of underlying illness
- Age
- Inappropriate antibiotic therapy
- Shock
- Bilateral pulmonary infiltrates
- Prior antibiotic therapy
- Neoplastic disease
- Duration of prior hospitalization
- Supine head position in patients being ventilated

gram-negative bacilli and *Staphylococcus aureus* (Table 6.2). Oropharyngeal colonization with aerobic gram-negative bacilli is unusual or of short duration in healthy, nonhospitalized individuals. However, in moderately ill patients, the carriage rate increases to 16% and reaches 57% in critically ill patients. With repeat cultures, colonization rates approach 75%. Severity of illness, longer duration of hospitalization, prior or concomitant use of antibiotics, advanced age and disability, poor nutrition, intubation and major surgery have all been identified as factors associated with gram-negative oropharyngeal colonization.

TABLE 6.2 — RISK FACTORS ASSOCIATED WITH OROPHARYNGEAL COLONIZATION

- Severity of illness
- Prolonged hospitalization
- Prolonged stay in intensive-care unit
- Advanced age
- Antibiotic therapy
- Endotracheal intubation
- Tracheostomy
- Gastric acid-suppressing therapy
- Major surgery
- Malnutrition
- Smoking
- Preexisting lung disease
- Uremia

Many risk factors have been identified for the development of nosocomial pneumonia, especially in ventilated patients (Table 6.3). Endotracheal intubation breaches most of the natural barriers in the upper airway. It impairs mucociliary clearance and injures the epithelial surface, predisposing to attachment of organisms to the surface of the lower respiratory tract. The endotracheal tube may become encrusted with a biofilm containing microorganisms. This may

TABLE 6.3 — RISK FACTORS FOR NOSOCOMIAL PNEUMONIA IN VENTILATED PATIENTS

- Duration of mechanical ventilation
- Chronic lung disease
- Severity of illness
- Age
- Severe head trauma or presence of intracranial pressure monitor
- Barbiturate therapy after head trauma
- Gastric acid-inhibitor therapy or elevated gastric pH
- Gross aspiration of stomach contents
- Reintubation or self-extubation
- Upper abdominal or thoracic surgery
- Ventilator circuit changes at intervals less than 48 hours
- Supine head position
- Fall or winter season
- Prior antibiotic therapy
- Use of nasogastric tube
- Bronchoscopy
- Shock
- Emergency endotracheal intubation after trauma
- Blunt trauma
- Stress ulcer with bleeding

be dislodged into the lung and serve as a source of infection.

The role of the stomach as a potential reservoir for pathogens is controversial. Several studies have reported similar organisms in the stomach and trachea in patients developing nosocomial pneumonia. However, gastric colonization preceding upper airway colonization has only been demonstrated in a minority of patients. Bacteria multiply rapidly in the presence of an ileus or impaired gastric acidification. Histamine type 2 blockers and antacids have been identified as risk factors for nosocomial pneumonia, presumably because they encourage an environment in which bacteria can rapidly multiply. Some authors have suggested the use of sucralfate for stress ulcer prophylaxis in the intubated patient, but reduced rates of nosocomial pneumonia have not been consistently demonstrated.

Other less common means of acquiring pneumonia include inhalation of microorganisms, seeding from the bloodstream and reactivation of latent infection (tuberculosis). Aspiration in mechanically ventilated patients occurs around the outside of the endotracheal tube rather than through the lumen. Leakage around the endotracheal cuff can be demonstrated in most patients. Other sources of pathogens are aspiration from the stomach or the nose and paranasal sinuses. Nursing the patient in the semirecumbent position can minimize aspiration of gastric content, but oropharyngeal aspiration is not affected by this maneuver. Outbreaks of HAP have been reported with the use of contaminated mainstream nebulizers, cascade humidifiers, manual ventilation bags, spirometers and ventilator temperature probes. Frequent changes of ventilator circuits are also associated with an increased incidence of pneumonia. Poor infection control practices can lead to the transmission of pathogens by health-care providers. Rates of infection can be reduced by hand washing, a practice often ignored by nurses and, more frequently, by physicians.

Approach to Diagnosis

The diagnosis of VAP is difficult and the role of invasive testing is controversial. Clinicians are often confronted with a changing clinical or radiographic setting where specific therapy is demanded. While mainly relying upon clinical judgment, clinicians have made increasing use of what has been termed "invasive testing." Developed in 1987, several techniques have been developed to handle two problems:

- Contamination by the upper airway (by protecting the sampling fluid)
- Separation of infection from colonization (by using quantitative cultures).

However, concerns regarding diagnostic accuracy, reproducibility of results, diagnostic thresholds, nonstandardized methodology and lack of clinical outcome data have made the interpretation of clinical studies difficult.

The initial diagnosis of VAP depends upon clinical suspicion and the presence of new or progressive radiographic infiltrates. Clinical suspicion is triggered by the presence of some combination of fever, purulent tracheobronchial secretions and leukocytosis. This combination of findings is sensitive in predicting the presence of pneumonia in a group of patients preselected for suspected VAP but does not perform as well among unselected patients. If all three criteria are required along with a new or progressive lung infiltrate, the specificity for the diagnosis of VAP drops below 50%, which is clinically unacceptable.

The incidence of pneumonia in immunocompetent patients with a normal chest radiograph and a compatible clinical presentation (a common finding in immunocompromised patients with *Pneumocystis carinii* pneumonia) is unknown. The usual radiographic abnormalities are new or worsening infiltrates or air bronchograms. The sensitivity ranges from 50% to 78% for new or worsening infiltrates and 58% to 83% for air bronchograms. The reliability of chest radiographs is low, as there is only marginal reproducibility between two readers. These findings suggest that a combination of clinical criteria and radiographic abnormalities are useful screening tools for the presence of VAP, but other investigations may be required to confirm the diagnosis. Many noninfectious disorders may produce pulmonary infiltrates and fever, including:

- Congestive heart failure
- Atelectasis
- Adult respiratory distress syndrome
- Drug reactions
- Pulmonary embolism.

Other investigations that are routinely performed are blood cultures and thoracentesis of pleural fluid if a sample is obtainable. Blood cultures will be positive in 8% to 20% of all patients with HAP. Among patients with severe HAP, other sources of infection besides the lung are found in up to 50% of cases. Serologic studies searching for organisms such as *Mycoplasma pneumoniae*, *Chlamydia pneumoniae* and *Legionella* species are rarely performed since the results of these investigations take weeks to return, which is of no immediate help to the clinician.

Microscopic examination of endotracheal aspirates is the simplest noninvasive means of obtaining respiratory secretions from mechanically ventilated patients. It is an attractive option since it is readily performed at the bedside and requires few special skills. Using the standard criteria developed for assessment of Gram stain will produce a valid representation of the infectious organisms. Qualitative endotracheal aspirates usually identify organisms found by invasive tests, suggesting high sensitivity, but they frequently identify other nonpathogenic organisms, reducing the positive predictive value of the test. Sterile endotracheal aspirate cultures make the diagnosis of VAP unlikely.

The results of quantitative endotracheal aspirate cultures vary with the bacterial load, duration of ventilation and prior antimicrobial administration. The sensitivity of endotracheal aspirates ranges widely from 38% to 100%, while specificity ranges from 14% to 100%. Antibody coating of bacteria (a systemic response to infection) and the presence of elastin fibers (a means of detecting lung parenchymal destruction) are neither sensitive nor specific for the diagnosis of VAP.

Fiberoptic bronchoscopy allows direct sampling of the lower respiratory tract. However, the bronchoscope itself will be contaminated by organisms found in the upper airway. Sampling is usually performed in the distal airways where contamination is less likely. Bronchoalveolar lavage (BAL) involves the sequential instillation and aspiration of a large volume of saline through the distal port of the bronchoscope while it is wedged in a peripheral airway. BAL samples approximately 1 million alveoli if a standard 120-mL aliquot of saline is introduced into a pulmonary subsegment. The recovered material is examined for the presence of inflammatory cells, intracellular organisms and the percentage of squamous epithelial cells. Squamous epithelial cells signify upper airway contamination, while the presence of intracellular organisms in 2% or more of phagocytic cells indicates true bacterial infection. Quantitative cultures are performed and the presence of organisms in concentrations of 10^4 colony-forming units/mL is considered to be sufficient to confirm the diagnosis of pneumonia and identify the causative pathogen. The sensitivity of quantitative BAL fluid cultures ranges from 42% to 93% with a mean of 73%. This variability depends upon prior antibiotic treatment, type of study population and the reference test used. Previous antibiotic therapy reduces sensitivity.

Protected specimen brushing (PSB) involves a double-catheter brush system with telescoping cannulas and a distally occluding wax plug. The bronchoscope is inserted into a peripheral segment and the catheter is advanced beyond the tip of the bronchoscope. The inner cannula is advanced to eject the wax plug, and purulent secretions are sampled. The brush is retracted into the inner cannula, and the inner cannula is retracted into the outer cannula. Once the bronchoscope is removed, the brush can be advanced, cut with sterile wire cutters and placed in 1 mL sterile saline. Quantitative cultures are performed, and the presence of organisms in concentrations of 10^3 colony-forming units/mL is considered to be sufficient to confirm the diagnosis of pneumonia and identify the causative pathogen.

The sensitivity for PSB ranges from 33% to 100% with a median of 67%, and the specificity ranges from 50% to 100% with a median of 95%. Overall, PSB appears to be more specific than sensitive in diagnosing VAP. One of the difficulties associated with quantitative invasive techniques is the reproducibility of the test, especially around the diagnostic thresholds. The test properties vary directly with the cutoff points chosen, and some studies have indicated that the results vary when multiple samples are obtained.

Other techniques have been developed because of the inconvenience, expense and necessity of operator expertise and potential side effects of diagnostic testing using fiberoptic bronchoscopy. Blinded bronchial sampling (BBS) involves blindly wedging a catheter into a distal bronchus and then aspirating secretions but without instilling fluid. Mini-BAL usually employs a single-sheathed 50-cm sterile plugging telescoping catheter with the installation of 20 to 150 mL of lavage fluid. In some instances, an unprotected catheter is used. The blinded protected specimen brush (BPSB) incorporates a sterile brush, which is protected from contamination. None of these techniques have been standardized.

The sensitivity of BBS ranges from 74% to 97%, that of mini-BAL from 63% to 100%, and that of BPSB from 58% to 86%. The specificity ranges from

74% to 100% for BBS, from 66% to 96% for mini-BAL and from 71% to 100% for BPSB. In general, these ranges are similar to those reported for BAL and PSB. Side effects for blinded techniques appear to be minimal and, at worst, may be similar to those seen with fiberoptic bronchoscopy.

Several studies have indicated that management decisions based on the results of invasive tests as compared with empiric therapy or decisions based on the results of endotracheal aspirates lead to more frequent antibiotic changes but have no impact on mortality. On the other hand, withholding of antibiotics from patients when VAP is not confirmed by invasive tests is not associated with higher recurrence rates of VAP or increased mortality rates. The final decision to utilize invasive techniques or to base decisions on clinical criteria supplemented by the results of noninvasive microbiologic results resides with the individual physician. Local expertise, test availability and cost considerations must be taken into account.

SUGGESTED READING

Bonten MJ, Bergmans DC, Stobberingh EE, et al. Implementation of bronchoscopic techniques in the diagnosis of ventilator-associated pneumonia to reduce antibiotic use. *Am J Respir Crit Care Med*. 1997;156:1820-1824.

Boyce JM, Potter-Bynoe G, Dziobek L, Solomon SL. Nosocomial pneumonia in Medicare patients. Hospital costs and reimbursement patterns under the prospective payment system. *Arch Intern Med*. 1991;151:1109-1114.

Chastre J, Viau F, Brun P, et al. Prospective evaluation of the protected specimen brush for the diagnosis of pulmonary infections in ventilated patients. *Am Rev Respir Dis*. 1984;130:924-929.

Craven DE, Daschner FD. Nosocomial pneumonia in the intubated patient: role of gastric colonization. *Eur J Clin Microbiol Infect Dis*. 1989;8:40-50.

Craven DE, Steger KA. Nosocomial pneumonia in the intubated patient. New concepts on pathogenesis and prevention. *Infect Dis Clin North Am.* 1989;3:843-866.

El-Ebiary M, Torres A, González J, et al. Quantitative cultures of endotracheal aspirates for the diagnosis of ventilator-associated pneumonia. *Am Rev Respir Dis.* 1993;148(pt 1):1552-1557.

Fagon J, Chastre J, Hance A. Evaluation of clinical judgement in the identification and treatment of nosocomial pneumonia in ventilated patients. *Chest.* 1993;103:547-553.

Fagon J, Chastre J, Hance A, et al. Nosocomial pneumonia in ventilated patients. A cohort study evaluating attributable mortality and hospital stay. *Am J Med.* 1993;94:281-288.

Lambert RS, Vereen LE, George RB. Comparison of tracheal aspirates and protected brush catheter specimens for identifying pathogenic bacteria in mechanically ventilated patients. *Am J Med Sci.* 1989;297:377-382.

Luna CM, Vujacich P, Niederman MS, et al. Impact of BAL data on the therapy and outcome of ventilator-associated pneumonia. *Chest.* 1997;111:676-685.

Marik PE, Brown WJ. A comparison of bronchoscopic vs blind protected specimen brush sampling in patients with suspected ventilator-associated pneumonia. *Chest.* 1995;108:203-207.

Marquette CH, Copin MC, Wallet F, et al. Diagnostic tests for pneumonia in ventilated patients: prospective evaluation of diagnostic accuracy using histology as a diagnostic gold standard. *Am J Respir Crit Care Med.* 1995;151:1878-1888.

Marquette CH, Herengt F, Mathieu D, Saulnier F, Courcol R, Ramon P. Diagnosis of pneumonia in mechanically ventilated patients. Repeatability of the protected specimen brush. *Am Rev Respir Dis.* 1993;147:211-214.

Montravers P, Fagon JY, Chastre J, et al. Follow-up protected specimen brushes to assess treatment in nosocomial pneumonia. *Am Rev Respir Dis.* 1993;147:38-44.

Papazian L, Martin C, Meric B, Dumon JF, Gouin F. A reappraisal of blind bronchial sampling in the microbiologic diagnosis of nosocomial bronchopneumonia. A comparative study in ventilated patients. *Chest.* 1993;103:236-242.

Papazian L, Thomas P, Garbe L, et al. Bronchoscopic or blind sampling techniques for the diagnosis of ventilator-associated pneumonia. *Am J Respir Crit Care Med*. 1995;152(pt 1):1982-1991.

Sanchez-Nieto JM, Torres A, Garcia-Cordoba F, et al. Impact of invasive and noninvasive quantitative culture sampling on outcome of ventilator-associated pneumonia: a pilot study. *Am J Respir Crit Care Med*. 1998;157:371-376.

Shepherd KE, Lynch KE, Wain JC, Brown EN, Wilson RS. Elastin fibers and the diagnosis of bacterial pneumonia in the adult respiratory distress syndrome. *Crit Care Med*. 1995;23:1829-1834.

Souweine B, Veber B, Bedos JP, et al. Diagnostic accuracy of protected specimen brush and bronchoalveolar lavage in nosocomial pneumonia: impact of previous antimicrobial treatments. *Crit Care Med*. 1998;26:236-244.

Timsit JF, Misset B, Goldstein FW, Vaury P, Carlet J. Reappraisal of distal diagnostic testing in the diagnosis of ICU-acquired pneumonia. *Chest*. 1995;108:1632-1639.

Torres A, Martos A, Puig de la Bellacasa J, et al. Specificity of endotracheal aspiration, protected specimen brush, and bronchoalveolar lavage in mechanically ventilated patients. *Am Rev Respir Dis*. 1993;147:952-957.

Torres A, Puig de la Bellacasa J, Xaubet A, et al. Diagnostic value of quantitative cultures of bronchoalveolar lavage and telescoping plugged catheters in mechanically ventilated patients with bacterial pneumonia. *Am Rev Respir Dis*. 1989;140:306-310.

Wunderink RG, Woldenberg LS, Zeiss J, Day CM, Ciemins J, Lacher DA. The radiologic diagnosis of autopsy-proven ventilator-associated pneumonia. *Chest*. 1992;101:458-463.

Wunderink RG, Russell GB, Mezger E, Adams D, Popovich J Jr. The diagnostic utility of the antibody-coated bacteria test in intubated patients. *Chest*. 1991;99:84-88.

6

7 Management of Nosocomial Pneumonia

The outcome of nosocomial pneumonia can be improved with early, appropriate empiric therapy. Several studies have demonstrated that mortality rates for hospital-acquired pneumonia (HAP) are higher if the initial antimicrobial therapy was inadequate as demonstrated by subsequent invasive culture results. There is also evidence to suggest that if the initial empiric choice is incorrect, subsequent correction to a more appropriate choice does not improve the mortality rate in patients with ventilator-associated pneumonia (VAP). It appears that in severely ill patients, the initial empiric therapy is the most important decision a physician can make.

An approach to the management of these patients that has gained wide acceptance includes an assessment of the severity of illness and risk factors that may predispose the patient to specific respiratory pathogens. Categorizing patients in this manner allows identification of likely pathogens and renders the choice of antimicrobials more rational. This approach has been used in a Canadian statement on the initial management of HAP. Subsequently, the recently published American Thoracic Society statement on initial therapy for HAP expands upon the Canadian document by adding the time of onset of the illness as another variable to be considered.

Enteric gram-negative bacilli and *Staphylococcus aureus* are the bacterial pathogens most commonly associated with HAP (Table 7.1). In patients with VAP, several reports have suggested that the infection may be polymicrobial. Bacterial pathogens predominate

TABLE 7.1 — MICROBIOLOGY OF NOSOCOMIAL PNEUMONIA

- Bacterial (80% to 90%):
  - Gram-negative bacilli (50% to 70%):
    - *Pseudomonas aeruginosa*
    - Enterobacteriaceae
  - *Staphylococcus aureus* (15% to 30%)
  - Anaerobic bacteria (10% to 30%)
  - *Haemophilus influenzae* (10% to 20%)
  - *Streptococcus pneumoniae* (10% to 20%)
  - *Legionella* species (4%)
- Viral (10% to 20%):
  - Cytomegalovirus
  - Influenza
  - Respiratory syncytial virus
- Fungal (< 1%)

in this clinical setting, but viral and fungal pneumonia occurs occasionally. Viral pneumonia occurs in the hospital setting, but the diagnosis is often missed because there are few unique clinical features to separate it from bacterial pneumonia, and the appropriate investigations (viral cultures, viral serology, rapid viral antigen tests) are rarely ordered. Viral pathogens should be considered during epidemic nosocomial infections, especially if there is a concomitant community outbreak.

Another approach which is helpful is to consider the likely pathogens according to the time after hospitalization that pneumonia developed (Table 7.2). Among patients with early-onset pneumonia (occurring within the first 5 days of hospitalization) relatively simple-to-treat organisms predominate. In contrast, late-onset pneumonia is usually characterized by infection with more resistant organisms.

A core group of bacterial pathogens has been identified. These organisms are common in all groups of patients and need to be covered in all circum-

TABLE 7.2 — ORGANISMS ASSOCIATED WITH EARLY- AND LATE-ONSET HOSPITAL-ACQUIRED PNEUMONIA

Early-Onset Pneumonia
- Enteric gram-negative bacilli:
  – *Escherichia coli*
  – *Klebsiella* species
  – *Proteus* species
  – *Serratia marcescens*
- *Haemophilus influenzae*
- Methicillin-sensitive *Staphylococcus aureus* (MSSA)
- *Streptococcus pneumoniae*

Late-Onset Pneumonia
- *Acinetobacter* species
- Methicillin-resistant *Staphylococcus aureus* (MRSA)

stances. Among these core organisms are enteric gram-negative bacilli such as *Enterobacter* species, *Escherichia coli*, *Klebsiella* species, *Proteus* species, and *Serratia marcescens* (Table 7.3). *Haemophilus influenzae* and gram-positive organisms, including methicillin-sensitive *S aureus* (MSSA) and *Streptococcus pneumoniae*, may also be identified. Multiresistant gram-negative organisms such as *Pseudomonas aeruginosa* do not fall into the category of core organisms.

TABLE 7.3 — CORE ORGANISMS

- Enteric gram-negative rods:
  – *Enterobacter* species
  – *Escherichia coli*
  – *Klebsiella* species
  – *Proteus* species
  – *Serratia marcescens*
- *Haemophilus influenzae*
- Methicillin-resistant *Staphylococcus aureus* (MRSA)
- *Streptococcus pneumoniae*

The definition of severe HAP has been adapted from that used for severe community-acquired pneumonia (CAP) (Table 7.4). Any patient residing in the intensive-care unit (ICU) or being admitted to the ICU falls into this category. Other factors that have been designated include the presence of:

- Respiratory failure
- Rapid radiographic progression
- Multilobar pneumonia
- Cavitation of a lung infiltrate
- Evidence of severe sepsis with hypotension
- End-organ damage.

Patients should be classified according to the severity of illness, the presence of specific risk factors for pathogens and the time of onset of the illness in relation to the day of hospital admission. This allows patients to be divided into three major groups:

TABLE 7.4 — DEFINITION OF SEVERE HOSPITAL-ACQUIRED PNEUMONIA

- Admission to the intensive-care unit
- Respiratory failure (need for mechanical ventilation or FiO_2 requirement > 35% to maintain oxygen saturation > 90%)
- Rapid radiographic progression, multilobular pneumonia or cavitation of lung infiltrate
- Evidence of severe sepsis with hypotension and/or end-organ dysfunction:
  – Shock (systolic BP < 90 mm Hg or diastolic BP < 60 mm Hg)
  – Requirement for vasopressors for more than 4 h
  – Urine output < 20 mL/h or total urine output < 80 mL in 4 h
- Acute renal failure requiring dialysis

Abbreviations: FiO_2, forced inspiratory oxygen; BP, blood pressure.

- Patients without unusual risk factors who present with mild-to-moderate HAP at any time during hospitalization or severe HAP of early onset (Tables 7.5 and 7.6).
- Patients with specific risk factors with onset at any time during hospitalization and patients with severe HAP either of early onset with specific risk factors or of late onset (Table 7.7).
- Patients without unusual risk factors who present with severe HAP of late onset or severe HAP of early onset if risk factors are present (Table 7.7).

The usual pathogens associated with mild-to-moderate pneumonia occurring at any time during hospitalization in patients without risk factors include enteric gram-negative bacilli such as *Enterobacter* species, *E coli*, *Klebsiella* species, *Proteus* species, and *S marcescens*. Other important pathogens in this group which need to be covered include *H influenzae*, *S pneumoniae* and MSSA; these are the core pathogens. For patients infected with these, a second- or nonpseudomonal third-generation cephalosporin (cefuroxime or ceftriaxone), a fourth-generation cephalosporin (cefepime) or a β-lactam/β-lactamase inhibitor combination (ampicillin/sulbactam, ticarcillin/clavulanate, or piperacillin/tazobactam) should suffice (Table 7.5). In penicillin-allergic patients, a fluoroquinolone or clindamycin/aztreonam combination are reasonable alternatives. In the event of a suspected *Pseudomonas* infection, combination therapy is always recommended.

Therapeutic Options

Despite previous teaching, there is no convincing linkage between presenting symptoms, findings on physical examination or laboratory test results and

TABLE 7.5 — ONSET OF MILD-TO-MODERATE HOSPITAL-ACQUIRED PNEUMONIA ANY TIME DURING HOSPITALIZATION IN PATIENTS WITH NO UNUSUAL RISK FACTORS OR EARLY ONSET OF SEVERE HOSPITAL-ACQUIRED PNEUMONIA

Core Oganisms	Core Antibiotics

• Enteric gram-negative bacilli:
  – *Enterobacter* species
  – *Escherichia coli*
  – *Klebsiella* species
  – *Proteus* species
  – *Serratia marcescens*
• *Haemophilus influenzae*
• Methicillin-resistant *Staphylococcus aureus*
• *Streptococcus pneumoniae*
	• Second- or nonpseudomonal third-generation cephalosporin (cefuroxime or ceftriaxone)
	• Fourth-generation cephalosporin (cefepime)
	• β-Lactam/β-lactamase inhibitor combination (ampicillin/sulbactam, ticarcillin/clavulanate, or piperacillin/tazobactam)
	• If patient is allergic to penicillin:
	  – Fluoroquinolone (ciprofloxacin, if not *S pneumoniae*)
	  – Clindamycin/aztreonam combination

TABLE 7.6 — ONSET OF MILD-TO-MODERATE HOSPITAL-ACQUIRED PNEUMONIA ANY TIME DURING HOSPITALIZATION IN PATIENTS WITH RISK FACTORS

Core Organisms Plus	Core Antibiotics Plus
• Anaerobes: – Recent abdominal surgery – Witnessed aspiration	Clindamycin or β-lactam/β-lactamase inhibitor alone
• *Staphylococcus aureus:* – Coma – Head trauma – Diabetes mellitus – Renal failure	± Vancomycin (until methicillin-resistant *Staphylococcus aureus* excluded)
• *Legionella* species: – High-dose corticosteroids	Macrolide ± rifampin
• *Pseudomonas aeruginosa:* – Prolonged intensive-care unit stay – Corticosteroids – Prior antibiotics – Structural lung disease	Treat as severe hospital-acquired pneumonia

7

139

TABLE 7.7 — EARLY ONSET OF SEVERE HOSPITAL-ACQUIRED PNEUMONIA DURING HOSPITALIZATION IN PATIENTS WITH RISK FACTORS OR LATE ONSET OF SEVERE HOSPITAL-ACQUIRED PNEUMONIA WITH NO RISK FACTORS

Core Oganisms Plus	Therapy
Pseudomonas aeruginosa *Acinetobacter* species	Aminoglycoside or ciprofloxacin plus one of the following: • Antipseudomonal penicillin • Cefepime or cefoperazone • Imipenem or meropenem • Aztreonam (only for gram-negatives)
Consider methicillin-resistant *Staphylococcus aureus*	± Vancomycin

specific pathogens. Thus microbiologic techniques have been developed to permit recognition of the causative pathogen. It would be preferable to identify the pathogen since such identification makes optimal antimicrobial selection possible. This is particularly relevant in this era of increasing antimicrobial resistance. Knowledge of the pathogen also limits the consequences of antibiotic abuse, including:

- Higher costs
- Increased resistance
- Adverse drug reactions.

Identifying pathogens of potential epidemiologic significance such as *Legionella* or inducible β–lactamase-producing Enterobacteriaceae would have a profound effect on antimicrobial selection and outcome. In comparison to the total costs of hospitalization, the costs associated with diagnostic testing are relatively trivial.

Unfortunately, the results of diagnostic testing have not proved to be sufficiently reliable to make therapeutic decisions. Several studies have indicated that there is reasonable concordance between clinical and microbiologic criteria for pneumonia. Some investigators have argued that antibiotic treatment is indicated in most cases with intermediate likelihood of pneumonia and in all cases with high likelihood, even if low colony counts are found. Only in low-risk patients with mild impairment can the delay in antimicrobial treatment while awaiting the results of invasive testing be justified. In the only randomized, prospective clinical trial comparing invasive techniques versus noninvasive techniques for the management of patients with VAP, invasive techniques led to more frequent antibiotic changes with no change in the mortality rate.

Empiric treatment has been recommended for the treatment of CAP by two carefully drafted guidelines, while the most recent guideline in this area has stressed the importance of pathogen-directed therapy. In the management of HAP, two North American guidelines recommended an empiric approach similar to that recommended for CAP. Knowledge of the usual microbial etiologies for HAP makes antimicrobial selection relatively simple. Factors that predict unusual pathogens, such as severity of illness or previous use of antimicrobials, should be identified.

The time of onset of pneumonia in relation to the day of admission helps predict microbiology. Early-onset VAP (defined as occurring during the first 4 days of the hospital stay) is often caused by *S pneumoniae*, *H influenzae*, *Moraxella catarrhalis* and, uncommonly, anaerobes. These are community-acquired pathogens and the pneumonia is a reflection of infection that has been incubating in the community but presents early in the course of hospitalization. Late-onset pneumonia (occurring more than 3 to 4 days after admission) is commonly caused by enteric gram-negatives, including *P aeruginosa*, *Acinetobacter* or *Enterobacter* species, or by *S aureus*.

Monotherapy vs Multidrug Therapy

Single-agent therapy with β-lactams, first-generation cephalosporins or macrolides is not feasible simply because these agents do not have a sufficiently broad spectrum of activity. In general, clinicians have relied upon combination antibiotic therapy to ensure broad coverage and to prevent the emergence of resistant organisms.

Aminoglycosides demonstrate good activity against the target pathogens but, unfortunately, as agents for nosocomial pneumonia, exhibit significant flaws. Aminoglycoside levels in pulmonary secretions are 10% to 45% of simultaneously measured serum aminoglycoside levels. Since toxic side effects limit the dosing capabilities of the aminoglycosides, levels achievable in respiratory tissues may be inadequate to eradicate most Enterobacteriaceae. Aminoglycosides perform poorly in an acidic environment with an eightfold reduction in antibacterial activity at pH 6.4 when compared with its activity at pH 7.4. The acidic environment associated with pneumonia, particularly in areas of necrosis or abscess, may inactivate aminoglycosides.

Several randomized controlled trials have demonstrated an association between the use of synergistic antibiotic combinations and improved therapeutic outcomes. However, many broad-spectrum antibiotics can cover the usual pathogens associated with nosocomial pneumonia. Initial therapy should cover the enteric gram-negative organisms and *S aureus*. Among the antibiotics which are active against these pathogens are:

- Third-generation cephalosporins:
  - Ceftazidime
  - Ceftriaxone
  - Cefotaxime
  - Cefoperazone
- Fourth-generation cephalosporins:
  - Cefepime
  - Cefpirome
- Older fluoroquinolones:
  - Ciprofloxacin
- Newer fluoroquinolones:
  - Levofloxacin
  - Sparfloxacin
  - Trovafloxacin
- Carbapenems:
  - Imipenem/cilastatin
  - Meropenem
- An extended spectrum β-lactam/β-lactamase inhibitor:
  - Ticarcillin/clavulanate
  - Piperacillin/tazobactam.

Among these, only ceftazidime, cefepime, cefpirome, imipenem/cilastatin, meropenem and ciprofloxacin would be considered to be active against *P aeruginosa*. Clinical efficacy of single-drug empiric therapy for nosocomial pneumonia has generally been equivalent to combination regimens. However, reports of efficacy in nosocomial pneumonia should not be extrapolated to pneumonia caused by *P aeruginosa* simply because most of these studies have not included enough patients infected with this organism to definitively demonstrate equivalence. Other problems that have been identified with single-agent therapy include emergence of antibiotic-resistant bacteria while on therapy and, occasionally, development of serious bacterial superinfections.

Problems With Drug-Resistant Organisms

■ Methicillin-Resistant *S aureus*

Staphylococci have been identified as important agents associated with community- and hospital-acquired infections for decades. In 1968, the first large outbreak of methicillin-resistant *S aureus* (MRSA) infections in the United States was reported at the Boston City Hospital. Once established in institutions, MRSA is difficult to eradicate. It currently accounts for up to 50% of all nosocomial *S aureus* isolates. Infections due to MRSA commonly occur in surgical and critically ill patients. The National Nosocomial Infection Surveillance System identified *S aureus* as the second most common pathogen after *P aeruginosa* causing nosocomial pneumonia. Recent adult community-acquired cases have followed influenza in more than half the cases and were associated with a 30% crude mortality rate.

The identified risk factors for this infection include increased length of stay and previous antibiotic therapy. Compared with other etiologies of nosocomial pneumonia, patients who are infected with *S aureus* are more likely to be less than 25 years of age, in coma, not users of corticosteroids and have antecedent trauma. Using a step-forward logistic regression analysis, only coma is defined as significantly influencing the development of *S aureus* pneumonia. Other investigators have identified neurosurgical patients, especially those treated for cerebral edema, and burn patients are at increased risk for *S aureus* pneumonia. Patients who develop MRSA have a different profile than those infected with MSSA. MRSA-infected patients are more likely to:

- Be older than 25 years of age
- Have received corticosteroids before developing infection
- Have been ventilated more than 6 days
- Have received antibiotics
- Have had preceding chronic obstructive lung disease compared with patients infected with MSSA.

The presence of bacteremia, septic shock and mortality is higher in the MRSA group. Hematogenous spread of *S aureus* to the lungs has been reported in patients with right-sided endocarditis, in users of illicit intravenous drugs, and in those with skin and soft-tissue infection, burns, pyomyositis and infected intravenous catheters. Transmission of MRSA is related to transient carriage on the hands of hospital personnel.

In MSSA infections, the semisynthetic penicillins are the most active agents. These include methicillin, oxacillin, and nafcillin. Other useful agents include an extended-spectrum β-lactam/β-lactamase inhibitor (ticarcillin/clavulanate, ampicillin/sulbactam, piperacillin/tazobactam) and the cephalosporins. The first- and second-generation cephalosporins (cefazolin, cefuroxime) are more potent than the third-generation cephalosporins against MSSA. The treatment of choice for MRSA is still vancomycin. Alternatives to vancomycin are few, but include teicoplanin, trimethoprim/sulfamethoxazole (in limited cases) and the new streptogramins. RP59500 (quinupristin/dalfopristin) is composed of two streptogramins, A and B, which act synergistically to inhibit protein synthesis. The efficacy of these new agents is currently being investigated.

■ Multi–Drug-Resistant Gram-Negative Rods

With the introduction of the β–lactamase-stable cephalosporins (second- and third-generation), stable, multiresistant, derepressed mutants of gram-negative bacteria have emerged during therapy. Failure of therapy or relapse after discontinuation of therapy has been reported with these agents. These organisms have been responsible for hospital outbreaks even in patients not receiving the cephalosporins.

These inducible β-lactamases are chromosomally mediated and not related to plasmids. In normal circumstances, these enzymes are repressed, which leads the casual observer to conclude that the organisms are sensitive to the tested antibiotics (usually cephalosporins or other stable β-lactams). However, with exposure to a β-lactam, increased levels of β-lactamases are produced, leading to resistance to multiple β-lactam antibiotics and clinical failures. The nonfastidious gram-negative bacilli that possess inducible β-lactamases include *Enterobacter* species (most commonly), *Serratia* species, *Citrobacter freundii*, *Proteus* species, *Providencia* species, *Morganella* species and *P aeruginosa*. In this case, simple exposure to a cephalosporin may lead to rapid emergence of resistance. When *Enterobacter* species are isolated from clinical samples, it may be prudent to avoid third-generation cephalosporins regardless of *in vitro* susceptibility. Resistance has emerged in 14% to 56% of treated patients, while the combination of clinical failure and resistance has been identified in 7% to 30% of patients. Emergence of resistance is seen more often with treatment of respiratory tract and bone and soft-tissue infections than with infections of the urinary tract.

The addition of another drug such as an aminoglycoside or another β-lactam has not prevented the emergence of resistance. Several studies have suggested that there is good correlation between the use of second- and third-generation cephalosporins and the occurrence of multiresistant gram-negative bacilli. Selective pressure leads to the emergence of resistance, but these organisms have a propensity for secondary spread within an institution. Early detection of these strains, judicious use of the cephalosporins and the use of barrier precautions in infected patients are necessary to prevent widespread hospital outbreaks. Consideration of a different class of antimicrobials, including fluoroquinolones, may be indicated.

Patients With Specific Risk Factors With Onset During Hospitalization

In patients at risk for anaerobic infection (recent abdominal surgery, witnessed aspiration), the addition of clindamycin to the usual second- or third-generation cephalosporin is recommended (Table 7.6). A β-lactam/β-lactamase inhibitor combination or a new fluoroquinolone with anaerobic activity (moxifloxacin) could be selected as a single agent. While aspiration is the common mechanism leading to the development of pneumonia, gross aspiration leading to anaerobic lung infection is uncommon. There are almost no data for the use of an antibiotic with anaerobic activity for pneumonia in the absence of lung necrosis or abscess formation.

In individuals at increased risk for *S aureus* infection (those with coma, head trauma, diabetes mellitus, renal failure), the possibility of methicillin resistance drives the consideration of vancomycin in addition to the core antibiotics. Among patients at risk for infection with *Legionella* species (eg, those who have received high-dose corticosteroids), a macrolide or a fluoroquinolone with or without rifampin should be considered.

Patients With Severe HAP (Early Onset With Specific Risk Factors or Late Onset)

Patients with severe HAP with risk factors or patients with late-onset pneumonia should be initially treated with broad-spectrum antibiotics that will cover multiresistant pathogens such as *P aeruginosa* or *Acinetobacter* species (Table 7.7). A regimen consisting of an aminoglycoside or ciprofloxacin plus one of an antipseudomonal penicillin, β-lactam/β-lactamase inhibitor, cefpirome or cefoperazone, imipenem or meropenem should be selected.

In the best randomized prospective trial of severe pneumonia, ciprofloxacin was compared with imipenem as single-agent therapy. Ciprofloxacin-treated patients had a higher bacteriologic eradication rate and a higher clinical response rate. When *P aeruginosa* was recovered from initial respiratory tract cultures, failure to achieve bacteriologic eradication and development of resistance during therapy were common in both groups. This study demonstrated that monotherapy for severe pneumonia is safe and effective but that other agents are required if *P aeruginosa* is suspected. The new fluoroquinolones do not have the same activity as ciprofloxacin against *P aeruginosa* and would not add anything to the standard recommended therapy.

These recommendations are for initial empiric management of patients with HAP. Once the pathogen is identified or a good clinical response is obtained, therapy can be simplified. In the only randomized, prospective clinical trial comparing invasive techniques with noninvasive techniques for the management of patients with VAP, invasive techniques led to more frequent antibiotic changes with no change in the mortality rate. It remains unclear whether routine follow-up microbiologic investigations are required. Certainly, in patients failing to respond to the initial empiric regimen, further investigations and a reexamination of the antibiotic selection is required.

SUGGESTED READING

American Thoracic Society. Hospital-acquired pneumonia in adults: diagnosis, assessment of severity, initial antimicrobial therapy, and preventive strategies. A consensus statement. *Am J Respir Crit Care Med.* 1996;153:1711-1725.

Chow JW, Fine MJ, Shlaes DM, et al. *Enterobacter* bacteremia: clinical features and emergence of antibiotic resistance during therapy. *Ann Intern Med.* 1991;115:585-590.

Fink MP, Snydman DR, Niederman MS, et al. Treatment of severe pneumonia in hospitalized patients: results of a multicenter, randomized, double-blind trial comparing intravenous ciprofloxacin with imipenem-cilastatin. The Severe Pneumonia Study Group. *Antimicrob Agents Chemother.* 1994;38:547-557.

Kollef MH. Ventilator-associated pneumonia. *Chest.* 1994;106:646. Letter.

LaForce FM. Systemic antimicrobial therapy of nosocomial pneumonia: monotherapy versus combination therapy. *Eur J Clin Microbiol Infect Dis.* 1989;8:61-68.

Mandell LA, Marrie TJ, Niederman MS and the Canadian Hospital Acquired Pneumonia Consensus Conference Group. Initial antimicrobial treatment of hospital acquired pneumonia in adults: a conference report. *Can J Infect Dis*. 1993;4:317-321.

Sanchez-Nieto JM, Torres A, Garcia-Cordoba F, et al. Impact of invasive and noninvasive quantitative culture sampling on outcome of ventilator-associated pneumonia: a pilot study. *Am J Respir Crit Care Med*. 1998;157:371-376.

8 Switch and Step-Down Therapy

In our current health-care environment, hospitals and physicians are challenged to provide a high standard of care in a more efficient way. An expert panel of the American Thoracic Society has confronted this challenge by formulating practice guidelines based on a review of data on community-acquired pneumonia (CAP) accessed from recent literature. By attempting to standardize the care of such patients, the CAP practice guidelines sought to improve clinical management. Hospitals and other health-care organizations have used these guidelines to streamline care and reduce cost. Recommended strategies include limiting diagnostic procedures, such as routine Gram stain and fiberoptic bronchoscopy. The issues of duration of antibiotic therapy and timing of switch from intravenous (IV) to oral medications were left deliberately vague.

As the pressures of cost containment have increased, the appropriate duration of IV antibiotics and hospital stay and the cost of antibiotic therapy have come under scrutiny. More data are becoming available that stress innovative nontraditional approaches to the antibiotic management of CAP such as home IV treatment and therapy with oral antibiotics. Early administration of antibiotic therapy either at home, in the clinician's office, or in the emergency department has been associated with improved survival in pneumonia. It is becoming clear that a substantial portion of hospitalized CAP patients can be safely switched to oral antibiotics earlier in their hospital course without any untoward events.

Definitions

Replacing IV antibiotics with effective oral antibiotics in the treatment of serious infections (eg, CAP, nosocomial pneumonia, urinary tract infections) is known as *switch therapy* (see *Approach to Switch Therapy* this chapter). If the change is accomplished with the same antibiotic as the IV antibiotic (eg, erythromycin), then it is labeled *step-down therapy*. If a different drug is used (eg, switching from an IV third-generation cephalosporin to oral erythromycin), then this approach is defined as *sequential therapy*. The clinical concept is identical, however, switching to oral antibiotics with similar or identical bacterial spectrums.

Because data on this subject are still emerging, a standard of care has yet to be firmly established. Nevertheless, several authors have shown that the institution of switch therapy may be both safe and associated with economic benefits. The common theme that links these is the identification of low-risk patients who are responding clinically to IV therapy.

Switch therapy has several potential benefits. From the patient perspective, switch therapy may have clinical and psychological benefits. Among these are decreasing nosocomial infection (ie, urinary tract and catheter-related infections) and length of hospital stay, thereby allowing the patient early discharge for full recovery at home. From the physician's point of view, switch therapy may allow for a more focused approach to patient care with an emphasis on clearly definable clinical endpoints. Health-care organizations may benefit from switch therapy by allowing the care of CAP patients to be standardized and streamlined. Clinical practice guidelines may be formulated that facilitate management of CAP at reduced cost. These potential benefits need to be evaluated in further prospective studies.

Other potential benefits of switching to oral antimicrobials for CAP include decreased complications of IV therapy, such as thrombophlebitis, line sepsis and decreased incidence of nosocomial infections. Most patients believe their quality of life would be improved by switching to oral antibiotics and earlier discharge from the hospital. These theoretic benefits, although intuitively obvious, are of unknown significance and await prospective evaluation.

Factors That Influence Antimicrobial Therapy

Determining the type, duration and switch to oral therapy is complicated by the fact that in the majority of patients with CAP, no pathogen has been identified. Even when carefully sought, a putative pathogen is documented in one half or less of cases of CAP. Therefore, in most instances, a specific microbiologic diagnosis is not established and the physician uses empiric antibiotics based on epidemiologic data. When an etiologic pathogen is identified (either initially or at a later time), then the antibiotic spectrum can be narrowed. When no pathogen is discovered, empiric antibiotics are continued.

Several factors play a role in deciding when to switch from IV to oral antibiotics in CAP. These include:
- Patient factors
- Pathogen characteristics
- Antibiotic properties.

■ **Patient Factors**

Patient factors that have traditionally influenced antibiotic decisions include:
- Severity of illness
- Clinical characteristics:
  - Patient age

- Comorbid medical illness
- Medical status
- Vital sign abnormalities
- Pulmonary and nonpulmonary organ dysfunction
- Laboratory abnormalities:
  - White blood cell count
  - Arterial blood gas abnormalities
  - Elevated blood urea nitrogen levels
  - Bacteremia
- Radiographic patterns:
  - Parapneumonic effusion
  - Abscess formation.

Multilobar infiltrates or radiographic progression must also be taken into account in making this decision.

■ Pathogen Characteristics

Pathogen characteristics that impact on the route and duration of therapy include:

- Virulence patterns
- Resistance patterns
- Whether the pathogen is intracellular or extracellular.

For example, a virulent and resistant pathogen causing CAP, such as methicillin-resistant *Staphylococcus aureus*, usually necessitates a more prolonged course of IV antibiotics as compared with pneumonia caused by the less virulent and more antibiotic sensitive *Mycoplasma pneumoniae*.

■ Antibiotic Properties

Antibiotic properties that allow initiation of switch therapy include:

- Antimicrobial spectrum
- Dosing schedule
- Bioavailability

- Patient tolerance to the antibiotic
- Expense.

All of these listed properties influence compliance. The characteristics of the ideal oral antibiotic used in switch therapy would be one that has:
- Identical antimicrobial spectrum to that of the IV antibiotic
- Once- or twice-a-day dosing to improve compliance
- High level of bioavailability
- No adverse side effects
- Low acquisition cost
- Few drug/drug interactions.

Approach to Switch Therapy

8

The data available on the use of switch therapy in CAP are limited. Several studies evaluating its safety and efficacy are available. In one, Weingarten and colleagues (1996) applied a switch-therapy practice guideline retrospectively to 503 hospitalized patients with CAP. The practice guideline was based upon three criteria that were used to categorize patients as being low risk on hospital day 3. These three criteria were:
- No obvious reason for continued hospitalization (eg, hypoxia)
- Absence of a high-risk pneumonia pathogen (eg, *S aureus*)
- No life-threatening complications during hospitalization (eg, acute myocardial infarction).

Based on this practice guideline, these investigators reported that only 33% of patients met their criteria retrospectively at day 3 for switch to oral antibiotics. The authors reported that the quality of care would not have been affected in 98.2% of the patients had they been switched to oral therapy on day 3. If these same patients were discharged from the hospital on day 4, 93.4% of them would have had no change in their quality of care. Given the retrospective application of the practice guideline, it is impossible to draw any definite conclusions from these data.

In another study, 120 patients admitted to the hospital with CAP were evaluated prospectively for switch therapy. In this study, patients were treated initially with IV ceftizoxime 1 g every 12 or 24 hours. Switch therapy with oral cefixime 400 mg once daily was initiated if patients met the following criteria:

- Resolution of fever
- Improved cough and respiratory distress
- Improved leukocytosis
- Presence of normal gastrointestinal tract absorption.

Of the 120 patients studied, 45 (37.5%) were not considered candidates for switch therapy. The 75 patients who met switch-therapy criteria received IV antibiotics for a mean of 3 days prior to receiving oral medication. There were no significant differences in length of therapy or clinical outcome between the different IV regimens in this study. Switch-therapy failure rate necessitating readmission to the hospital was 1.3%, indicating a 98.7% clinical cure rate. Of the patients treated with this switch-therapy protocol, none had any untoward effects, including the one patient who was readmitted to the hospital and treated with IV erythromycin with good response. The authors also estimated that $104,524 were saved since the patient stayed in the hospital for 4 days rather than the usual 6 days.

The same practice guideline was prospectively applied in another study with an alternative month design (no intervention in the first month of the study, intervention in the second month of the study, no intervention in the third month of the study, etc). If patients were enrolled in the study during a noninterventional month (controls), data were collected, but no active interventions were initiated by the study team. If patients were enrolled in the study during an interventional month, data were also collected, but a team of case-management nurses, pharmacists, and physicians were instructed to inform the attending physician of the guideline recommendations.

Of the 717 hospitalized patients with a pneumonia-related diagnosis over the 22-month study period, 146 patients (20.4%) were considered at low risk and candidates for the switch-therapy practice guidelines. Adherence to the practice guideline occurred in 76% of cases during the interventional months. Of considerable interest was the fact that during the noninterventional months (the times when control patients were enrolled), 69% of the cases adhered to the practice guideline. The authors suggest that this occurred because physicians may have been sensitized to the practice guideline during both the interventional and noninterventional months. The severity of pneumonia was relatively low as evidenced by the 30-day mortality rate of 0.7% (predicted 9%). This study suggests that switch-therapy practice guidelines aimed at both early conversions from IV antibiotics to oral therapy and early hospital discharge are feasible and safe in carefully selected patients.

In summary, this suggests that patients hospitalized for CAP can be switched to oral antimicrobials when there is evidence of clinical improvement on IV antibiotics and when patients have no associated risk factors for increased morbidity and mortality (Table 8.1) However, several caveats are worth considering. Patients hospitalized for CAP have varying coexisting medical diseases and are managed by physicians with different practice patterns. There is inherent variability in the patient-physician interaction, resulting

8

TABLE 8.1 — FACTORS ASSOCIATED WITH INCREASED MORBIDITY AND MORTALITY

- Postsplenectomy state
- Chronic alcohol abuse
- Altered mental status
- Vital sign abnormalities:
  - Respiratory rate > 30
  - Systolic BP < 90 mm Hg
  - Diastolic BP < 60 mm Hg
  - Temperature > 38.3° C (101° F)
- PaO_2 < 60 mm Hg
- $PaCO_2$ > 50 mm Hg
- Need for mechanical ventilation
- Metastatic (extrapulmonary) infection
- WBC < 4000 or > 30,000/mm^3
- Renal dysfunction, eg BUN > 20 mg/dL
- Unfavorable chest radiographic patterns:
  - Multilobular infiltrates
  - Effusions
  - Rapidly progressive infiltrates
  - Cavitation
- Evidence of severe infection:
  - Metabolic acidosis
  - DIC
  - Severe sepsis or septic shock
  - ARDS

Abbreviations: BP, blood pressure; PaO_2, partial pressure of arterial oxygen; $PaCO_2$, partial pressure of carbon dioxide in arterial gas; WBC, white blood cell [count]; BUN, blood urea nitrogen; DIC, disseminated intravascular coagulation; ARDS, acute respiratory distress syndrome.

in a wide range of diagnostic approaches and initial antibiotic regimens. It is therefore impossible to establish a set formula for switch therapy. This concept is further complicated by the fact that not all patients are created equal. Patients respond to therapy at different rates as influenced by the interaction of types and severity of preexisting morbidities, age, severity of pneumonia and pathogen virulence. Factors that contribute to slowly resolving or nonresolving pneumonia are also important since they impact on response to therapy (Table 8.2). It seems likely that response assessment must be ongoing rather than attempting to set predetermined time intervals for conversion to oral therapy. This hypothesis, however, remains to be tested.

TABLE 8.2 — FACTORS THAT CAN SLOW PNEUMONIA RESOLUTION

- Increased age
- Alcohol abuse
- Significant coexisting disease
- Severe pneumonia
- Multilobular disease
- Infection with a virulent pathogen such as:
  – *Legionella pneumophila*
  – *Staphylococcus aureus*
  – Gram-negative bacilli
- History of smoking
- Persistent leukocytosis and fever
- Bacteremic infection

Based on the current data, switch therapy may be instituted if certain criteria are met (Table 8.3).

Antibiotic Principles

In most patients with CAP no pathogen has been identified, even after extensive diagnostic testing. In this common clinical situation, empiric antibiotics are continued. If the pathogen is identified, the antibiotic regimen can be narrowed. In either scenario, the patient should be evaluated for switch to oral antibiotics once clinical improvement and factors associated with increased morbidity and mortality are absent (Table 8.1).

TABLE 8.3 — CRITERIA USED TO IDENTIFY CANDIDATES FOR STEP-DOWN THERAPY

- Intact gastrointestinal absorption
- Improving cough
- Improving respiratory distress
- Declining temperature
- Absence of high-risk or resistant pathogens, eg, *Staphylococcus aureus*
- Absence of unstable coexisting disease
- Absence of complications, eg, congestive heart failure
- Improving leukocytosis

The oral antibiotic chosen for switch therapy should encompass the same antibacterial spectrum as the IV agent. In addition, the oral regimen should have a good dosing schedule and a low adverse-reaction profile to ensure completion of therapy. The dosing schedule is of particular importance since this affects patient compliance. Using an oral antibiotic with a frequent dosing schedule is associated with reduced compliance and potential medication error than when using one with a once- or twice-a-day dosing regimen.

No one antibiotic regimen has yet been shown to have definitive superiority to another in switch therapy. Knowledge of local epidemiology and resistance patterns should guide both the initial IV empiric therapy and the subsequent oral antibiotic. For example, if a patient is treated with an IV second- or third-generation cephalosporin, and no pathogen is identified, switch therapy may be initiated with an oral second- or third-generation cephalosporin. If the patient is treated initially with an intravenous β-lactam/β–lactamase-inhibitor combination and no pathogen is identified, switch therapy may be initiated with an oral β-lactam/β–lactamase-inhibitor combination (amoxicillin/clavulanate). In the case of a patient initially treated with an IV macrolide, switch therapy can be either with an oral erythromycin or with one of the newer macrolides that have less-complex dosing regimens. Studies favoring the newer macrolides suggest better compliance, fewer side effects and similar clinical cure rates. If a specific pathogen is identified, switch to an oral antibiotic that covers that pathogen is necessary. For example, if penicillin-sensitive *Streptococcus pneumoniae* is identified in the blood, oral penicillin may be appropriate.

Summary

There are three treatment options available for patients hospitalized with CAP. The first option, the traditional one, is to initiate therapy with parenteral antibiotics and continue them for the entire course. The second option is the switch-therapy option, starting with IV antibiotics and then changing to oral therapy to complete treatment. Finally, physicians may use oral antibiotics from the outset, depending on the initial severity of the infection. Data on this latter treatment option are limited and more information will become available in the near future, especially when some of the newer antibiotics used to treat CAP become available, specifically the newer fluoroquinolones.

Step-down therapy is not only the initiation of oral antibiotics. Appropriate candidates must be identified and timing ascertained for the change over. Predetermining conversion time (eg, day 3 switches) should be replaced with the practice of ongoing evaluation (Figure 8.1). Prospective controlled studies are needed to validate the hypothetical benefits and limited risk of switch therapy for CAP (Table 8.3).

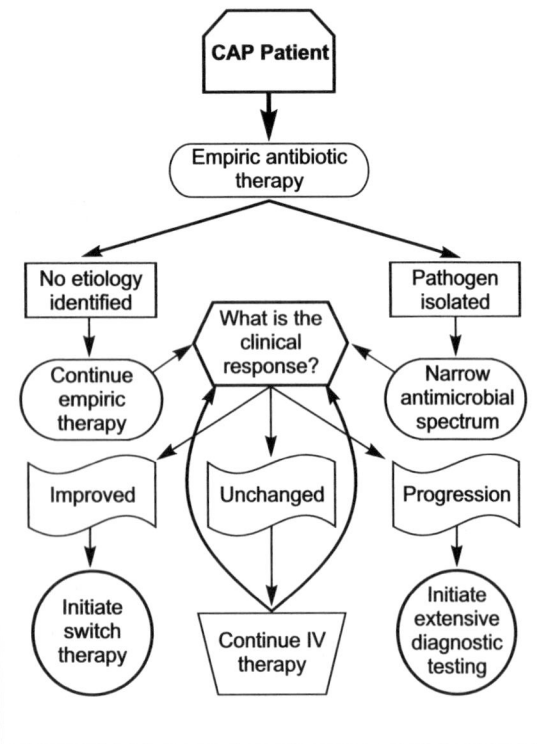

FIGURE 8.1 — DIAGRAM OUTLINING THE MANAGEMENT OF PATIENTS WITH COMMUNITY-ACQUIRED PNEUMONIA

CAP Patient

Empiric antibiotic therapy

No etiology identified → Continue empiric therapy → Improved → Initiate switch therapy

What is the clinical response?

Unchanged → Continue IV therapy

Pathogen isolated → Narrow antimicrobial spectrum

Progression → Initiate extensive diagnostic testing

Abbreviation: CAP, community-acquired pneumonia.

SUGGESTED READING

American Thoracic Society. Guidelines for the initial management of adults with community-acquired pneumonia: diagnosis, assessment of severity, and initial antimicrobial therapy. *Am Rev Respir Dis*. 1993;148:1418-1426.

Briceland LL, Nightingale CH, Quintiliani R, Cooper BW, Smith KS. Antibiotic streamlining from combination therapy to monotherapy utilizing an interdisciplinary approach. *Arch Intern Med*. 1988;148:2019-2022.

British Thoracic Society and the Public Health Laboratory Service. Community-acquired pneumonia in adults in British hospitals in 1982-1983: a survey of aetiology, mortality, prognostic factors and outcome. *Q J Med*. 1987;62:195-220.

Hendrickson JR, North DS. Pharmacoeconomic benefit of antibiotic step-down therapy: converting patients from IV ceftriaxone to oral cefpodoxime proxetil. *Ann Pharmacother*. 1995;29:561-565.

Ramirez JA, Srinath L, Ahkee S, Huang A, Raff MJ. Early switch from IV to oral cephalosporins in the treatment of hospitalized patients with community-acquired pneumonia. *Arch Intern Med*. 1995;155:1273-1276.

Weingarten SR, Riedinger MS, Hobson P, et al. Evaluation of a pneumonia practice guideline in an interventional trial. *Am J Respir Crit Care Med*. 1996;153:1110-1115.

Weingarten SR, Riedinger MS, Varis G, et al. Identification of low-risk hospitalized patients with pneumonia. Implications for early conversion to oral antimicrobial therapy. *Chest*. 1994;105:1109-1115.

8

9 Natural History of Pneumonia

Introduction

Pneumonia that fails to respond to treatment is a common problem. Although quantification of the frequency of this problem is difficult, approximately 15% of pulmonary consultations and 8% of bronchoscopies are done to evaluate nonresolving pneumonia. In the intensive-care unit, up to 90% of patients will have persistent radiographic infiltrates on chest x-ray (CXR). Clinicians are confronted with a complex challenge when this occurs.

It is difficult to define:
- What is normal resolution
- What is delayed resolution
- What is progression of disease.

A specific pathogen cannot be identified in up to 50% of cases of community-acquired pneumonia (CAP), and two or more etiologies are identified in up to 5% of cases. This leads to significant diagnostic uncertainty when patients fail to respond to empiric therapy. As a result, when pneumonia fails to respond to treatment, the question becomes whether the diagnosis of pneumonia is even correct, since many conditions can mimic pneumonia.

Thus the first step in evaluating nonresolving pneumonia is to discriminate between normal and nonresolving pneumonia in order to avoid unnecessary diagnostic tests. This requires an understanding of the pathophysiology of pneumonia resolution. Once nonresolving pneumonia is identified, the second step is a systematic consideration of infectious and noninfectious etiologies. Finally, an approach to diagnosis and management must be developed based on the differential diagnosis.

Pathophysiology

The difficulty in defining the nonresolving pneumonia syndrome is that the normal resolution of pneumonia is not a clearly defined process. Given this uncertainty, it is useful to consider the resolution of pneumonia as a spectrum including:

- Normal resolution
- Slowly resolving pneumonia
- Progressive pneumonia.

The parameters used to describe this spectrum include both clinical and radiographic criteria.

Clinical criteria that have been studied include (Table 9.1):

- Fever
- Cough
- Crackles
- White blood cell count
- PaO_2 level
- C-reactive protein.

TABLE 9.1 — RATE OF RESOLUTION OF PHYSICAL AND LABORATORY ABNORMALITIES	
Abnormalities	**Duration (d)**
Fever	2 to 4
Cough	4 to 9
Crackles	3 to 6
Leukocytosis	3 to 4
C-reactive protein	1 to 3

Subjective response is usually noted within 3 to 5 days of starting treatment. Most studies of resolution of pneumonia have not focused on symptoms but have instead focused on radiographic resolution. Investigators have usually not defined normal resolution but have instead defined slowly resolving pneumonia. Investigators differ slightly in their definition of slow resolution, but in most instances slowly resolving pneumonia has been defined by the persistence of radiographic abnormalities for greater than 1 month in a clinically improved host.

Although the ideal transition point for defining slowly resolving pneumonia varies, from a clinical standpoint the critical distinction lies in differentiating pneumonias that are progressive from those that are merely slow to resolve. The latter can be observed without further testing, while the former requires further investigation. The clinical decision that a patient has nonresolving and progressive pneumonia must take into account factors that affect the expected rate of resolution. These factors include:

- Comorbidities
- Age
- Severity
- Type of infectious agent.

■ **Comorbidities and Resolution of Community-Acquired Pneumonia**

Pneumonia frequently occurs in patients with comorbidities that may delay the resolution of pneumonia (Table 9.2). While patients without these comorbidities will usually demonstrate clearing of radiographic infiltrates by 4 weeks, only 20% to 30% of patients with these comorbidities will clear by 4 weeks. The frequency of these comorbidities increases with age and thus concurrent comorbidities are more common in the elderly. As an example, in patients less than 50 years of age, chronic obstructive

TABLE 9.2 — Comorbidities Associated With Delayed Resolution of Pneumonia

Condition	Pathophysiology
Chronic obstructive pulmonary disease	Impaired cough and mucociliary clearance
Alcoholism	Aspiration, malnutrition, impaired immune function
Neurologic disease	Aspiration, impaired clearance of secretions
Coronary heart disease	Edema fluid, impaired lymphatic drainage
Renal failure	Hypocomplementemia, impaired macrophage and neutrophil function, reduced humoral immunity
Malignancy	Impaired immune function, altered colonization
Human immunodeficiency virus	Impaired cell-mediated and humoral immunity
Diabetes mellitus	Impaired neutrophil function and cell-mediated immunity

pulmonary disease (COPD) is present in 5% of CAP cases. In patients older than 50 years of age, COPD is present in more than 30% of CAP cases.

■ Age and Resolution of Community-Acquired Pneumonia

Despite the concurrence of comorbidities and advanced age, several studies have demonstrated that age itself is an independent risk factor for delayed clearing. Approximately 90% of patients younger than 50 years of age show radiographic resolution by 4 weeks. In contrast, only 30% of patients older than 50 years of age without concurrent disease will have radiographic resolution by 4 weeks. Thus age is among the most important factors associated with delayed resolution.

■ Severity and Resolution of Community-Acquired Pneumonia

In addition to being associated with comorbidities, age is also associated with an increased risk for more severe pneumonia. However, severity of disease remains an independent risk factor for delayed resolution. The time to radiographic resolution for severe CAP has been estimated at 10 weeks, as compared with 3 to 4 weeks for mild-to-moderate pneumonia. Definitions of normal resolution vary significantly in the literature, in part because of wide variations in the severity of illness triggering admission. This has an impact on the expected normal rate of resolution, since severity impacts on the rate of resolution.

■ Infectious Agents and Resolution of Community-Acquired Pneumonia

The rate of radiographic and clinical improvement also varies with the infectious agent (Table 9.3). This section will focus on the features that are relevant to

TABLE 9.3 — INFECTIOUS AGENT AND RATE OF RESOLUTION

Infectious Agent	Initial CXR Deterioration	CXR Clearing	Residual Abnormalities
Legionella species	Majority	2 to 6 mo	25%
Staphylococcus aureus	Majority	3 to 5 mo	Common
Streptococcus pneumoniae sepsis	Majority	3 to 5 mo	25% to 35%
Streptococcus pneumoniae (nonbacteremic)	Occasional	1 to 3 mo	Rare
Gram-negative	Occasional	3 to 5 mo	10% to 20%
Haemophilus influenzae	Occasional	1 to 5 mo	Occasional
Chlamydia species	Rare	1 to 3 mo	10% to 20%
Mycoplasma pneumoniae	Rare	2 to 4 wk	Rare
Moraxella catarrhalis	Rare	1 to 3 mo	Unusual

Abbreviation: CXR, chest x-ray.

resolution of pneumonia with respect to the most common microorganisms. These include *Streptococcus pneumoniae*, *Chlamydia pneumoniae*, *Haemophilus influenzae*, and *Legionella* and *Mycoplasma* species.

Streptococcus pneumoniae

Pneumococcal pneumonia accounts for up to 65% of CAP infections, and therefore accounts for most cases of infectious nonresolving pneumonia syndromes. It is also the best studied of the infectious etiologies in terms of the rate of resolution and the factors that affect resolution. In normal individuals without predisposing illnesses, clinical improvement precedes radiographic improvement.

Clinical improvement is relatively rapid in uncomplicated cases. When auscultation was the primary tool for assessing response to therapy, clinicians were able to detect abnormal findings on physical examination in only 8% of patients at 1 month. Similarly, fever resolves rapidly, with only 6% of patients demonstrating fever beyond 20 days. Risk factors for delayed resolution of ausculatory findings and fever include more severe presentation and multilobar disease.

In contrast, radiographic improvement is often much slower. Despite relatively rapid clinical improvement, anywhere from 20% to 30% of patients will have no improvement on CXR at 1 week. Indeed, initial worsening of the CXR is common. Risk factors for delayed radiographic resolution include:

- Bacteremia
- Persistent fever or leukocytosis beyond 6 days
- Age greater than 50 years
- COPD
- Alcoholism.

Radiographic clearing occurs by 1 to 3 months in non-bacteremic cases and in 3 to 5 months in bacteremic cases. Residual radiographic abnormalities are rare in nonbacteremic cases but are present in up to 35% of bacteremic cases.

Legionella pneumophila

Legionella is increasingly recognized as an important pathogen in patients with severe CAP. *Legionella* is one of the three most frequent etiologic agents that cause rapidly progressive pneumonias. It is frequently encountered in the compromised host and in the elderly, with established risk factors for infection with *Legionella* being:

- Cigarette use
- Alcoholism
- Age greater than 65
- Immunosuppression with corticosteroids
- Dialysis
- Marrow transplantation.

Many of these predisposing conditions are likewise risk factors for delayed resolution, so it is not surprising that the rate of resolution for *Legionella* infection is slower than that for other organisms.

Ninety percent of *Legionella* infections are due to *Legionella pneumophila*, and 80% of these are due to serogroup 1. Thus, most of the literature on the natural history of *Legionella* infections is based on this one serogroup. As in pneumococcal infections, clinical improvement precedes radiographic improvement. The radiographic infiltrates and clinical picture are usually indistinguishable from severe pneumococcal infections. There is usually an initial patchy infiltrate that subsequently becomes confluent and even bilateral, often despite appropriate antibiotic therapy.

The distinguishing features of *Legionella* infections are the:

- Propensity for initial radiographic deterioration
- Prolonged resolution of radiographic infiltrates

- Prolonged convalescence associated with this infection.

Radiographic deterioration occurs in up to two thirds of patients infected with *Legionella*, as compared with 4% of patients with nonbacteremic pneumococcal pneumonia. In addition, after this initial deterioration, resolution is slower than with pneumococcal infections. Radiographic clearing only begins after 2 to 3 weeks, with 50% being abnormal at 10 weeks. Resolution may take as long as 6 to 12 months, with residual fibrosis being evident in up to 25% of patients. Even after radiographic resolution, generalized weakness and fatigue may persist for months. In the initial description of Legionnaires' disease in Philadelphia, patients frequently complained of fatigue and shortness of breath when surveyed up to 2 years after the event, with half demonstrating residual abnormalities on pulmonary function testing.

Mycoplasma pneumoniae

Mycoplasma pneumoniae is a common cause of respiratory tract infections; however, it is a relatively rare cause of severe pneumonia. Clinically apparent pneumonia occurs in only 3% to 13% of patients infected, with most patients being young adults. *Mycoplasma* accounts for approximately 5% of hospital pneumonias but is unusual in those older than 65 years of age. Because these infections generally are less severe and occur in a younger population, it is not surprising that the rate of resolution is faster than with other types of pneumonia.

The initial radiographic pattern is one of interstitial infiltrates, with progression to air space disease with consolidation. Multilobar involvement is common, occurring in 50% to 60% of cases. Radiographic deterioration on treatment is rare, occurring in less than 25% of cases. Acute respiratory distress syndrome is a rare complication of *Mycoplasma* pneumonia, with only 10% of patients requiring mechanical ventilation.

In contrast to Legionnaires' disease, rapid resolution of *Mycoplasma* pneumonia is common. There is usually a rapid clinical improvement that occurs in the first 2 weeks, in part reflecting the predominantly young population affected. Average duration of radiographic abnormalities is 2 to 4 weeks, depending on the use of antibiotics. Forty percent have complete radiographic resolution at 4 weeks and 90% at 8 weeks. Residual scarring and fibrosis are rare.

Chlamydia pneumoniae

Chlamydia pneumoniae infection is common, with 30% to 50% of young adults having serologic evidence of infection. Distinguishing features of *Chlamydia* infection include:
- Increased frequency of hoarseness
- Lack of fever
- Prolonged period before seeking medical attention
- Extrapulmonary manifestations, including:
  - Erythema nodosum
  - Encephalitis
  - Guillain-Barré syndrome.

The disease is relatively mild and mortality is rare, with prompt resolution being the rule in younger patients. However, relapse is common when erythromycin is given for only 2 weeks, and it is therefore advisable to treat with either 3 weeks of erythromycin or 2 weeks of a tetracycline. Radiographically, *Chlamydia* pneumonia is indistinguishable from other forms of pneumonia, with lobar and interstitial infiltrates being common. Initial radiographic deterioration is rare, with radiologic clearing requiring 1 to 3 months. Resolution is intermediate between *Myco-*

plasma and *Legionella*. Fifty percent of chest radiographs clear by 4 weeks, with up to 20% taking longer than 9 weeks. Residual radiographic scarring and fibrosis are seen in 10% to 20% of cases.

Haemophilus influenzae

Haemophilus influenzae has become an increasingly common cause of pneumonia and is now recognized as a common pathogen in the elderly, in hospitalized patients and in cigarette smokers. Risk factors for severe infection include:

- COPD
- Malignant disease
- Diabetes
- Alcoholism
- Immunosuppression.

In a surveillance study in Finland (Takala 1990), 71% of cases occurred in patients who were severely immunocompromised and 55% of invasive cases occurred in those over the age of 50. Invasive cases are more commonly caused by encapsulated strains, which are also associated with a higher risk for severe sepsis and mortality. Unencapsulated strains are less frequently associated with mortality but are more often associated with a prolonged febrile tracheobronchitis.

The clinical presentation of pneumonia caused by *Haemophilus* is not unique and it is therefore impossible to reliably differentiate it from other pneumonias, particularly that caused by pneumococcus. A multilobar pattern of bronchopneumonia with a pleural effusion is considered classic, but this finding is by no means specific.

The natural history of *Haemophilus* infection has not been well studied, and there are no distinguishing features regarding the rate of resolution. Based on its propensity to infect the immunocompromised and elderly, the rate of resolution can be expected to be slow.

Clinical improvement is also slow, with many patients being hospitalized for up to 2 to 3 weeks, with only half returning to their previous level of function by 6 weeks. Similarly, radiographic resolution can be expected to be slow relative to other pneumonias.

Pneumonia of Unknown Etiology

Because *S pneumoniae* and *L pneumophila* are both common in severe CAP, the normal resolution time for severe CAP may be expected to range from to 3 to 12 weeks. Since half of all pneumonias will have no isolated pathogen, it becomes clear that the possible upper limit of normal resolution will be quite high.

Based on these studies, it is apparent that the normal time to resolution for severe CAP has a broad distribution curve, depending upon a variety of factors. Many patients with nonresolving pneumonia will actually be within the limits of normal resolution once these other factors are taken into consideration. Those patients with slow radiographic resolution but a good clinical response can be defined as having slowly resolving pneumonia.

At some point in this spectrum, however, the patient crosses into the area of nonresolving pneumonia. Those patients with clinical deterioration under therapy can be defined as having progressive pneumonia. These two categories have significant overlap but are useful clinical definitions since patients with progressive disease are more likely to warrant additional diagnostic testing. Importantly, the term "pneumonia" in this situation does not necessarily equate with infection, since many patients with clinical deterioration may have a noninfectious disorder. Progressive disease in these cases may be due to factors associated with either infectious or noninfectious etiologies.

SUGGESTED READING

American Thoracic Society. Guidelines for the initial management of adults with community-acquired pneumonia: diagnosis, assessment of severity, and initial antimicrobial therapy. *Am Rev Respir Dis*. 1993;148:1418-1426.

Augustine G, Fein A, Feinsilver S, et al. When pneumonia fails to resolve: risk factors and diagnostic options and four questions to guide your evaluation. *J Crit Illness*. 1992;7:213-260.

Bartlett JG, Breiman RF, Mandell LA, File TM Jr. Community-acquired pneumonia in adults: guidelines for management. The Infectious Diseases Society of America. *Clin Infect Dis*. 1998;26:811-838.

British Thoracic Society. Guidelines for the management of community-acquired pneumonia in adults admitted to hospital. *Br J Hosp Med*. 1993;4:25.

British Thoracic Society and the Public Health Laboratory Service. Community-acquired pneumonia in adults in British hospitals in 1982-83: a survey of aetiology, mortality, prognostic factors and outcome. *Q J Med*. 1987;62:195-220.

Cunha BA. Clinical features of Legionnaires' disease. *Semin Respir Infect*. 1998;13:116-127.

Dietrich PA, Johnson RD, Fairbank JT, Walke JS. The chest radiograph in Legionnaires' disease. *Radiology*. 1978;127:577-582.

Fiore AE, Nuorti JP, Levine OS, et al. Epidemic Legionnaires' disease two decades later: old sources, new diagnostic methods. *Clin Infect Dis*. 1998;26:426-433.

Fang GD, Yu VL, Vickers RM. Disease due to Legionellaceae (other than *Legionella pneumophila*). Historical, microbiological, clinical, and epidemiological review [published erratum appears in *Medicine*. 1989;68:209]. *Medicine*. 1989;68:116-132.

Fang GD, Fine M, Orloff J, et al. New and emerging etiologies for community-acquired pneumonia with implications for therapy. A prospective multicenter study of 359 cases. *Medicine*. 1990;69:307-316.

9

Fein AM, Feinsilver SH, Niederman MS, Fiel S, Pai PB. When the pneumonia doesn't get better. *Clin Chest Med*. 1987;8:529-541.

Fein AM, Feinsilver SH, Niederman MS. Nonresolving and slowly resolving pneumonia. Diagnosis and management in the elderly patient. *Clin Chest Med*. 1993;14:555-569.

Fein AM, Feinsilver S, Niederman MS. Slowly resolving pneumonia in the elderly. In: Niederman MS, ed. *Respiratory Infections in the Elderly*. New York, NY: Raven Press; 1991:293-324.

Feinsilver SH, Fein AM, Niederman MS, Schultz DE, Faegenburg DH. Utility of fiberoptic bronchoscopy in nonresolving pneumonia. *Chest*. 1990;98:1322-1326.

Finnegan OC, Fowles SJ, White RJ. Radiographic appearances of *mycoplasma* pneumonia. *Thorax*. 1981;36:469-472.

Gleichman TK, Leder MM, Zahn DW. Major etiological factors producing delayed resolution in pneumonia. *Am J Med Sci*. 1949;218:309-320.

Grayston JT. *Chlamydia pneumoniae,* strain TWAR. *Chest*. 1989;95:664-669.

Grayston JT. *Chlamydia pneumoniae,* strain TWAR pneumonia. *Ann Rev Med*. 1992;43:317-323.

Helms CM, Viner JP, Sturm RH, Renner ED, Johnson W. Comparative features of pneumococcal, mycoplasmal, and Legionnaires' disease pneumonias. *Ann Intern Med*. 1979;90:543-547.

Israel HL, Weiss W, Eisenberg GM, et al. Delayed resolution of pneumonias. *Med Clin North Am*. 1956;40:1291-1303.

Jay SJ, Johanson WG J, Pierce AK. The radiographic resolution of *Streptococcus pneumoniae* pneumonia. *N Engl J Med*. 1975;293: 798-801.

Kirtland SH, Winterbauer RH. Slowly resolving, chronic, and recurrent pneumonia. *Clin Chest Med*. 1991;12:303-318.

Kroboth FJ, Yu VL, Reddy SC, Yu AC. Clinicoradiographic correlation with the extent of Legionnaires' disease. *Am J Roentgenol*. 1983;141:263-268.

Lattimer GL, Rhodes LV III, Salventi JS, et al. The Philadelphia epidemic of Legionnaires' disease: clinical, pulmonary, and serologic findings two years later. *Ann Intern Med.* 1979;90:522-526.

Lo CD, MacKeen AD, Campbell DR, Fraser DB, Marrie TJ. Radiographic analysis of the course of *Legionella pneumonia. J Can Assoc Radiol.* 1983;34:116-119.

Lowenkron SE, Niederman MS. Definition and evaluation of the resolution of nosocomial pneumonia. *Semin Respir Infect.* 1992; 7:271-281.

Macfarlane JT, Miller AC, Roderick Smith WH, Morris AH, Rose DH. Comparative radiographic features of community-acquired Legionnaires' disease, pneumococcal pneumonia, *Mycoplasma* pneumonia, and psittacosis. *Thorax.* 1984;39:28-33.

Marrie TJ. Normal resolution of community-acquired pneumonia. *Semin Respir Infect.* 1992;7:256-270.

Marrie TJ. Epidemiology of community-acquired pneumonia in the elderly. *Semin Respir Infect.* 1990;5:260-268.

Marrie TJ, Durant H, Yates L. Community-acquired pneumonia requiring hospitalization: 5-year prospective study. *Rev Infect Dis.* 1989;11:586-599.

Marrie TJ. Normal resolution of community-acquired pneumonia. *Semin Respir Infect.* 1992;7:256-270.

Marrie TJ, Grayston JT, Wang SP, Kuo CC. Pneumonia associated with the TWAR strain of *Chlamydia. Ann Intern Med.* 1987;106: 507-511.

McRae T. Delayed resolution in lobar pneumonia. *Johns Hopkins Hospital Rep.* 1910;15:277-280.

Mundy LM, Auwaerter PG, Oldach D, et al. Community-acquired pneumonia: impact of immune status. *Am J Respir Crit Care Med.* 1995;152:1309-1315.

Rodrigues J, Niederman MS, Fein AM, Pai PB. Nonresolving pneumonia in steroid-treated patients with obstructive lung disease. *Am J Med.* 1992;93:29-34.

9

Sullivan RJ Jr, Dowdle WR, Marine WM, Hierholzer JC. Adult pneumonia in a general hospital. Etiology and host risk factors. *Arch Intern Med*. 1972;129:935-942.

Takala AK, Eskola J, van Alphen L. Spectrum of invasive *Haemophilus influenzae* type b disease in adults. *Arch Inten Med*. 1990;150:2573-2576.

Torres A, Serra-Batlles J, Ferrer A, et al. Severe community-acquired pneumonia. Epidemiology and prognostic factors. *Am Rev Respir Dis*. 1991;144:312-318.

Zweig S, Lawhorne L, Post R. Factors predicting mortality in rural elderly hospitalized for pneumonia. *J Fam Pract*. 1990;30:153-159.

10

Possible Etiologies of Nonresolving Pneumonia

Infectious Etiologies

If the initial diagnosis of an infectious etiology is correct, factors that can lead to a progressive or nonresolving pneumonia need to be assessed. These factors include those associated with the:

- Pathogen
- Host
- Therapy.

■ Pathogen Factors

Alternative or unusual pathogens need to be considered in the patient who fails to respond to treatment. Although there is a potentially unlimited number of unusual pathogens that may cause nonresolving pneumonia, several warrant special attention (Table 10.1). Among these, the most important to consider are:

- Tuberculosis (TB) or other mycobacteria
- Fungi
- *Nocardia* and *Actinomyces*.

In addition, the possibility of a relatively common pathogen with resistance needs to be considered.

Tuberculosis

There has been an increase in the incidence of TB recently, and in certain populations, TB remains a significant concern. The suspicion of TB should be particularly high in:

- Immigrant populations

TABLE 10.1 — "UNUSUAL" PATHOGENS THAT CAN CAUSE NONRESOLVING PNEUMONIA

Pathogen (Related Disease)	Distinguishing Characteristics
Mycobacterium tuberculosis (tuberculosis)	High-risk populations, elderly
Atypical mycobacteria (bronchiectasis)	Positive acid-fast bacillus (AFB)
Nocardia (nocardiosis)	Immunocompromised host, positive AFB
Actinomyces israelii (actinomycosis)	Aspiration risk, chest wall involvement
Aspergillus (aspergillosis)	Immunocompromised host, vascular invasion
Endemic fungi: • *Histoplasma capsulatum* (histoplasmosis) • *Coccidioides immitis* (coccidioidomycosis) • *Blastomyces dermatitidis* (blastomycosis)	Appropriate travel history: • Mississippi River Valley • Southwestern United States • Southeast and midwest United States
Coxiella burnetii (Q fever)	Exposure to cats, cattle or sheep
Francisella tularensis (tularemia)	Exposure to rabbits or ticks

Chlamydia psittaci (psittacosis)	Avian sources
Yersinia pestis (plague)	Exposure to rats
Leptospira interrogans (leptospirosis)	Exposure to rats
Pseudomonas pseudomallei (melioidosis)	Southeast Asia (rodent exposure), mimics tuberculosis radiographically
Paragonimus westermani (paragonimiasis)	Asia/Africa/Central and South America
Hantavirus	Southwestern United States with exposure to mice
Anthrax	More common in Asia Minor, Iran, Turkey, Greece, South Africa; contact with infected animal carcasses or hides

- Patients with a history of intravenous drug abuse
- Patients with acquired immunodeficiency syndrome (AIDS) risk factors.

In addition, the elderly should also be considered at higher risk for TB, since the elderly still represent one of the largest repositories of TB in the United States. Infections in the elderly will usually represent reactivation disease, since the majority were infected 50 to 70 years ago. However, recent studies of epidemic spread in nursing homes indicate that new infections are also possible, so a high index of suspicion is necessary.

The clinical presentation of TB as a cause of nonresolving pneumonia will often be atypical, especially in the elderly. Atypical findings, such as nonspecific mid- or lower-lobe changes, are common. Similarly, up to one third of adult patients with newly diagnosed TB have atypical findings, irrespective of age. Thus the classic presentation of a cavitary infiltrate in the apical or posterior segments of one or both upper lobes may not always be present.

In this setting, the diagnosis of TB may be difficult. Tuberculin testing may be negative in 10% to 20% of patients with active disease and in an even higher percentage of the elderly and patients with AIDS. A two-step tuberculin test should be considered in the elderly to overcome this waning of delayed hypersensitivity. Sputum acid-fast cultures are positive in up to 80% of cases, but sputum is not always easy to obtain, especially in the elderly. Because culture results may take up to 6 weeks, newer methods, including the BAC-TEC culture system, are recommended to decrease the time needed to establish a diagnosis. Polymerase chain reaction testing has been approved for smear-positive specimens to allow confirmation of tuberculous disease, but its role in smear-negative patients remains to be determined.

Fungi

Both opportunistic as well as endemic fungi may mimic bacterial pneumonia. Of the opportunistic fungi, *Aspergillus* is the most important. The spectrum of pulmonary *Aspergillus* infections includes:

- Benign mycetomas
- Chronic necrotizing aspergillosis
- Invasive pulmonary aspergillosis.

Of these various forms, it is the chronic necrotizing and invasive forms that are most likely to be mistaken for bacterial pneumonia.

Chronic necrotizing aspergillosis represents a semi-invasive form of infection and is most commonly seen in the setting of preexisting chronic lung disease, often with chronic corticosteroid use. It may also be seen at the interface of a mycetoma and the normal lung. From a pathophysiologic standpoint, this syndrome represents the result of a host immune response that is barely able to hold the infection in check but which is not strong enough to eradicate it. The radiographic appearance is usually chronic and progressive, affecting the upper lobes more frequently.

Invasive aspergillosis is classically described as affecting neutropenic patients who have been on multiple antibiotics for several days. However, it is important to realize that aspergillosis is being increasingly recognized in two new groups of patients. The first group is the elderly with chronic lung disease who are on corticosteroids. In these cases, aspergillosis may mimic a bacterial infection, leading to significant delays in therapy. In one series, patients with invasive aspergillosis were treated an average of 18 days with multiple antibiotics before the diagnosis was made. In many of these cases, the diagnosis was only established postmortem.

The second new group at risk for *Aspergillus* infection is the AIDS population. Patients with advanced

AIDS are at increased risk for invasive aspergillosis. In addition, patients with less advanced disease (infection with the human immunodeficiency virus [HIV]) may develop one of three different patterns of tracheobronchitis that may mimic nonresolving pneumonia. These three patterns are:

- Obstructive bronchial aspergillosis
- Ulcerative tracheobronchitis
- Pseudomembranous tracheobronchitis.

Obstructive bronchial disease is characterized by thick mucous plugs filled with *Aspergillus* with little mucosal involvement. Ulcerative tracheobronchitis is characterized by additional mucosal and cartilaginous involvement. Pseudomembranous tracheobronchitis develops when there is extensive inflammation and invasion of the tracheobronchial tree with formation of a pseudomembrane of hyphae and necrotic debris. Thus in addition to the traditional neutropenic patient, the diagnosis of *Aspergillus* as a cause of nonresolving pneumonia should be considered in the elderly immunocompromised patient and in those with advanced AIDS.

The other major group of fungal infections that need to be considered as a cause of nonresolving pneumonia are the endemic fungi. The endemic fungi share many common clinical characteristics, but the most important element in establishing the diagnosis is a careful history, since each fungus can be found in certain geographic areas. *Histoplasma capsulatum* can be found in the Mississippi River valley, *Coccidioides immitis* in the southwestern United States and *Blastomyces dermatitidis* in the southeast and midwest United States. In the case of both histoplasmosis and coccidioidomycosis, most inhabitants will have immunologic evidence of prior exposure. Each of these fungi can cause a nonspecific acute febrile illness, which is usually self-limited and may easily be confused with community-acquired pneumonia (CAP).

The more difficult cases involve those patients who develop chronic and progressive disease. This usually involves the upper lobes and may be cavitary, often leading to a misdiagnosis of tuberculosis. Although blastomycosis is classically described as being masslike and coccidioidomycosis is described as producing thin-walled cavities, none of these fungi can be reliably separated on the basis of chest x-ray (CXR) findings.

In general, when the chest radiograph suggests TB but smears are negative for acid-fast organisms, these fungal infections should be considered. In addition, patients with HIV infection are at particularly high risk for disseminated infection with both histoplasmosis and coccidioidomycosis. Early consideration of these possibilities is essential in this group.

A combination of potassium hydroxide smear and culture of sputum may provide the diagnosis. Serology is generally not useful for histoplasmosis and blastomycosis. Immunoglobulin M (IgM) antibodies for coccidioidomycosis may be clinically useful and typically rise in the first 2 weeks, disappearing by the end of 1 month. Skin testing is available for histoplasmosis but is not useful since active infection cannot be distinguished from prior exposure and 90% of inhabitants in an endemic area can be expected to test positive. Although many experts believe skin testing is useful for coccidioidomycosis, a single skin test is not enough to document the onset of infection. It is therefore more useful to use skin testing as an epidemiologic tool rather than a specific diagnostic test in individual patients.

Nocardia and Actinomyces

Although *Nocardia* and *Actinomyces* are classified as higher order bacteria, both behave in a fashion more consistent with the pulmonary mycoses.

Both result in a chronic pulmonary disease that is difficult to diagnose because of the difficulty with isolating these pathogens. *Nocardia* can only be grown aerobically if cultures are kept and examined for up to 4 weeks, while *Actinomyces* requires strict anaerobic conditions with enriched media. Both are gram-positive organisms with branching filamentous pseudohyphae. *Nocardia* frequently stains positive on acid-fast smear, but *Actinomyces* is rarely positive. Because these organisms have relatively specific culture requirements and are difficult to stain, communication with the microbiology laboratory is essential when there is clinical suspicion of disease caused by either.

Patients with *Nocardia* infection present with a subacute or chronic condition, including cough, purulent sputum and night sweats. Infection frequently occurs in the setting of underlying malignancy or pulmonary alveolar proteinosis. Disseminated infection may occur, with the most serious consequence being central nervous system involvement with brain abscess. The most common radiographic presentation is that of a localized alveolar infiltrate that is usually homogenous, nonsegmental and often cavitary. Infection with *Actinomyces* has similar clinical and radiographic features, with the exception being the propensity of actinomycosis to extend across fissures and to involve the chest wall.

Resistant Pathogens

An important consideration in the approach to any pneumonia is the possibility of antibiotic resistance. In particular, the possibility of penicillin-resistant *Streptococcus pneumoniae* (PRSP) must be considered when evaluating patients with nonresolving pneumonia. PRSP was first described in the 1960s in Australia and New Guinea. In recent surveys from Europe, approximately 40% to 60% of pneumococci demonstrate intermediate- or high-level resistance. In the United States, resistance rates are lower but are rising, mimicking the trends seen previously in Europe. Among isolates of invasive pneumococcal disease, 25% to 50% of cases currently demonstrate penicillin resistance.

In patients with nonresolving pneumonia, it is reasonable to investigate the possibility of drug resistance as a possible contributing factor. The suspicion of PRSP should be especially high in cases of non-resolving pneumonia associated with risk factors for drug resistance. The risk factors for infection with PRSP include:

- Prior β-lactam therapy within 6 months
- Pneumonia within 1 year
- Hospitalization in the prior 3 months
- Nosocomial infection.

Of these factors, the most significant in univariate and multivariate analyses is prior β-lactam use, especially cephalosporins.

Once PRSP is either suspected or isolated, it becomes important to determine the level of penicillin resistance and the sensitivity pattern of the organism. The majority of PRSP strains have intermediate resistance to penicillin, defined as a minimum inhibitory concentration (MIC) > 0.1 and < 2.0 µg/mL. In the setting of intermediate resistance to penicillin, increasing the dose of penicillin to 12 to 18 million u/d is effective. Isolates with an MIC > 2 µg/mL are defined as having high-level resistance, and these cases should be treated with agents other than penicillin based upon their susceptibility testing.

Alternative agents include cefotaxime, ceftriaxone, imipenem, newer fluoroquinolones (grepafloxacin, levofloxacin, moxifloxacin), and vancomycin. Importantly, sensitivity patterns for cephalosporins do not necessarily follow penicillin-susceptibility patterns.

Pneumococcal isolates that have intermediate resistance to penicillin may have high-level resistance to cephalosporins. Therefore, sensitivity to cephalosporins and imipenem should be confirmed in cases of PRSP. Similarly, since macrolide resistance is less prevalent, these drugs may be useful alternatives, but their use still requires confirmation of sensitivity. If erythromycin resistance is demonstrated, clarithromycin, azithromycin and clindamycin should not be used, since there is significant cross-resistance. Newer fluoroquinolones, such as grepafloxacin, levofloxacin, and moxifloxacin, have demonstrated activity against PRSP and may be considered in cases of PRSP. Finally, vancomycin is the most reliable treatment for infection with PRSP since resistance to vancomycin has not yet been demonstrated. Vancomycin should be used in combination in all cases of PRSP meningitis.

■ Host Factors

The effect of various host factors, including comorbidities such as alcoholism, diabetes, chronic obstructive pulmonary disease (COPD), and age on the normal rate of resolution of pneumonia has been discussed previously (see Chapter 9, *Natural History of Pneumonia*). Most host factors cannot be altered and therefore do not necessarily impact directly on treatment. However, certain disorders of immune function warrant special attention because the underlying defect can be at least partially treated if recognized. These include AIDS and syndromes associated with deficiencies of humoral immunity.

Acquired Immunodeficiency Syndrome

With the experience gained from the HIV epidemic, most physicians are aware of *Pneumocystis carinii* pneumonia (PCP) as a cause of respiratory compromise in the HIV-infected patient. PCP was among the most common diseases associated with AIDS, being the initial manifestation in approximately two thirds of cases in older series. With the use of widespread prophylaxis, the dominance of PCP among the pulmonary pathogens associated with HIV has decreased, but it remains an important consideration. Bacterial pneumonia is now the most common initial lower respiratory tract infection in AIDS patients. Because of this, it is important to consider the possibility of HIV infection in patients with nonresolving pneumonia. If the diagnosis of unrecognized HIV is made, the spectrum of possible pathogens changes dramatically. The Infectious Disease Society of America recommends routine testing for HIV infection in patients with CAP between the ages of 15 and 54 occurring in hospitals where the rate of newly diagnosed HIV infection exceeds one case per 1000 discharges. Conditions that are much more likely in this setting and need to be considered in these cases include cryptococcal pneumonia, endemic fungi, TB and PCP.

Primary Humoral Immune Deficiencies

Primary humoral immune deficiencies are due to inherited defects in antibody production. While there are a huge number of diseases associated with secondary disorders of humoral or cellular immunity, the importance of identifying primary humoral immune deficiency syndromes lies in the fact that treatment with intravenous immune globulin (IVIG) has an effect on the incidence and resolution of pneumonia. The disorders most commonly associated with hypogammaglobulinemia in which IVIG is indicated include X-linked agammaglobulinemia, common variable immune deficiency (CVID), selective IgG subset deficiency and hypogammaglobulinemia with IgM.

All of these disorders are characterized by defects in the steps necessary for production of immunoglo-

191

bulins, from intrinsic defects within the B cell itself to problems with B cell/T cell interactions. The resulting deficiencies in immunoglobulin production lead to impaired opsonization and complement activation. Thus patients with relative or absolute hypogammaglobulinemia are prone to recurrent and refractory sinopulmonary tract infections with encapsulated organisms, leading to nonresolving pneumonias. Infections typically begin in infancy or early childhood so that most cases are recognized by the time patients reach adulthood. Importantly, certain disorders, most notably CVID and IgG subclass deficiency, may present in an atypical fashion at a later age. The most common pathogens in these patients include *Streptococcus pneumoniae* and *Haemophilus influenzae,* with *Mycoplasma* and *P carinii* being less common.

Monthly IVIG maintenance therapy markedly reduces the incidence and severity of pneumonia in these patients. Currently, protocols require maintenance infusions every 2 to 4 weeks to maintain a trough level of > 400 mg/dL. When patients with primary humoral immune deficiencies develop pneumonia, additional supplemental IVIG is warranted for treatment of the acute disease and facilitates resolution and decreases severity.

■ Therapy-Related Factors

When pneumonia fails to respond appropriately to treatment, certain aspects related to therapy need to be considered. These include consideration of possible medication errors as well as assuring adequate concentrations of antibiotics at the site of infection.

With respect to medication errors, it is especially important to carefully check dosing schedules, compliance and, when appropriate, drug levels. If intermediate-level resistant PRSP is present, higher doses of penicillin will be required as previously discussed.

Similarly, if PCP is suspected, higher doses of trimethoprim/sulfamethoxazole will be required. When aminoglycosides are used, it is important to check levels and adjust the dosing regimen accordingly. Similarly, as renal function changes, drug doses may require readjustment. In addition, since aminoglycosides do not penetrate the lung well, when utilizing a traditional dosing regimen it may be necessary to aim for higher peak concentrations, especially when treating infection caused by *Pseudomonas*. The effect of decreased pulmonary penetration on aminoglycoside efficacy using a once-daily dosing regimen has not yet been studied for pneumonia and remains unclear.

The other aspect of therapy is to guarantee that adequate levels of drug are reaching the site of infection by ruling out sequestered foci of infection. The two main forms of sequestered foci that may prevent adequate resolution of pneumonia are:

- Empyema
- Lung abscess.

Empyema evaluation can be facilitated by a variety of imaging techniques, including chest computed tomography (CT) and ultrasound. In the patient with nonresolving pneumonia, demonstration of any significant amount of pleural fluid should lead to consideration of a diagnostic thoracentesis to rule out empyema. Although the exact criteria for defining an empyema remain controversial, in the setting of a nonresolving or progressive pneumonia, it is prudent to aggressively evaluate all effusions for possible chest tube drainage. A pH less than 7.20, positive Gram stain, positive culture or demonstration of grossly purulent fluid should prompt chest tube placement.

Pulmonary abscesses are the other sequestered infectious foci that can lead to nonresolving pneumonia. Predisposing factors that should raise the suspicion of abscess formation include:

- Alcoholism
- Seizures
- Poor oral hygiene
- Previous aspiration.

A chest radiograph typically will demonstrate an air-fluid level, but a chest CT scan is more sensitive and can confirm the diagnosis in difficult cases. Because most patients with lung abscesses do well with only conservative management and a prolonged course of antibiotics, it is important to identify those factors associated with increased abscess-related mortality that may warrant a more aggressive approach. Factors that adversely affect the prognosis in patients with lung abscess include:

- Increased age
- Pediatric age
- Large cavity size
- Longer duration of symptoms prior to therapy
- Lower lobe location
- Association with malignant disease
- Multiple abscesses.

Intrabronchial aspiration is a contributing factor in fatal cases of lung abscess and has led to the recommendation that controlled drainage and improved physical measures be used to avoid intrabronchial spread. Thus although routine drainage is not necessary in all patients, in those at high risk and in those with nonresolving pneumonia, drainage should be considered.

A variety of techniques has been utilized to drain abscesses. These include:

- Bronchoscopic aspiration
- CT-guided aspiration
- Ultrasound guided aspiration.

However, some attempts at bronchoscopic aspiration have actually led to intrabronchial aspiration and acute respiratory distress syndrome (ARDS). Thus if bronchoscopic aspiration is considered, it should probably be limited to carefully selected patients in whom no other methods of drainage are possible. When bronchoscopy is done for either diagnostic or treatment purposes, there should be minimal use of depressant drugs and careful use of lidocaine to minimize the risk of intrabronchial spread.

Noninfectious Etiologies

Many noninfectious diseases may mimic pneumonia by presenting with persistent pulmonary infiltrates. The major categories of disease that warrant consideration as mimics of pneumonia include diseases that are (Table 10.2):
- Neoplastic
- Immunologic
- Drug induced
- Vascular.

10

■ Neoplastic
Neoplasms may cause a nonresolving pneumonia syndrome in one of two ways:
- By causing a postobstructive pneumonia or abscess
- By appearing as infiltrative processes with air bronchograms.

Neoplasms that cause postobstructive pneumonias and abscesses are most commonly bronchogenic carcinomas. Those that present as alveolar infiltrates include lymphoma and bronchoalveolar cell carcinoma.

TABLE 10.2 — NONINFECTIOUS ETIOLOGIES OF NONRESOLVING PNEUMONIA

Neoplastic
- Bronchogenic carcinoma
- Bronchoalveolar cell carcinoma
- Lymphoma

Immunologic
- Vasculitis:
  - Wegener's granulomatosis (WG)
  - Diffuse alveolar hemorrhage
- Bronchiolitis obliterans-organizing pneumonia (BOOP)
- Eosinophilic pneumonia syndromes:
  - Acute eosinophilic pneumonia
  - Chronic eosinophilic pneumonia
- Acute interstitial pneumonia
- Pulmonary alveolar proteinosis (PAP)
- Sarcoidosis

Drug Toxicity

Vascular
- Congestive heart failure (CHF)
- Pulmonary embolism

Bronchogenic Carcinoma

In cases of postobstructive pneumonia, the tumor occludes the bronchi either by endobronchial involvement or extrinsic compression. Bronchoscopy remains the method of choice for detecting endobronchial obstruction, since it allows for the simultaneous collection of biopsy and cytology specimens that are over 95% sensitive and specific for endobronchial malignancies. However, the overall frequency of endobronchial carcinoma as a cause of nonresolving pneumonia is surprisingly low, ranging from 0% to 8%. Despite this low prevalence, the relatively low risk of bronchoscopy makes it an appropriate consideration in those at especially high risk for lung cancer (eg, cigarette smokers older than 50 years of age).

Bronchoalveolar Cell Carcinoma

Bronchoalveolar cell carcinoma is traditionally characterized as a subtype of adenocarcinoma of the lung that is slow growing and frequently associated with the small peripheral airways and alveolar spaces. It may present as a focal alveolar infiltrate, often with air bronchograms, mimicking the radiographic appearance of pneumonia. Consolidation occurs in up to one third of cases, involving both segmental and lobar areas. Other radiographic appearances include pulmonary nodules and diffuse or multicentric alveolar infiltrates. The nodular form has a good prognosis, while the diffuse and multicentric forms have a worse prognosis.

Lymphoma

Lymphoma in the lung may present with focal alveolar infiltrates with air bronchograms, mimicking the radiographic appearance of pneumonia. When lymphoma affects the lung parenchyma, it may occur either as part of a systemic disease or as a true primary pulmonary lymphoma. Although lymphoma may initially present with radiographic evidence of pulmonary parenchymal involvement, it is rare, with only 10% of Hodgkin's and 4% of non-Hodgkin's lymphomas presenting with initial parenchymal pulmonary involvement. However, in both cases, as the disease progresses, lung involvement becomes progressively more common, rising to 38% of Hodgkin's and 24% of non-Hodgkin's cases. If pulmonary Hodgkin's is suspected, CT scan of the chest may be especially useful, since mediastinal lymphadenopathy is almost invariably present. Importantly, in cases of non-Hodgkin's lymphoma as well as Hodgkin's associated with HIV, mediastinal lymphadenopathy may be absent in up to 50% of cases.

■ Immunologic Diseases

Many immunologic diseases can be associated with some pulmonary manifestations, and it would be impossible to review each possible presentation that might mimic pneumonia. This discussion will focus on those that can present with an acute onset, have frequent pulmonary manifestations and be manifested with a paucity of extrapulmonary symptoms. These include:

- Systemic vasculitis
- Bronchiolitis obliterans-organizing pneumonia (BOOP)
- Eosinophilic pneumonia syndromes
- Acute interstitial pneumonia
- Pulmonary alveolar proteinosis
- Sarcoidosis.

Systemic Vasculitis

Fever, dyspnea and pulmonary infiltrates may be the initial manifestation of systemic vasculitis or a connective tissue disorder and may be easily mistaken for CAP. In most patients, extrapulmonary symptoms will be prominent and a prior history of vasculitis will be present. However, when extrapulmonary symptoms are lacking, differentiating pulmonary vasculitis from severe CAP may be difficult. Furthermore, patients with a previously established diagnosis of vasculitis are frequently on immunosuppressive agents for their vasculitis and are therefore prone to opportunistic infections. Distinguishing a nonresolving infectious process from worsening vasculitis can be especially difficult in these immunocompromised patients (Table 10.3).

Wegener's granulomatosis and the alveolar hemorrhage syndromes are the most frequent vasculitides to mimic pneumonia. Elevated serum antineutrophil cytoplasmic antibodies, acute renal insufficiency, rapidly filling hemoglobin or hemoptysis should suggest

TABLE 10.3 — ETIOLOGIES OF DIFFUSE ALVEOLAR HEMORRHAGE

Etiology	Distinguishing Characteristics
Goodpasture's syndrome	Anti-GBM antibodies
Connective tissue disorders	Most commonly lupus, ANA positive
Systemic vasculitis	Wegener's granulomatosis: c-ANCA positive Microscopic polyarteritis: p-ANCA positive
Drug toxicity	History of drug exposure, usually chemotherapeutic agents
Mitral stenosis	Diastolic murmur, history of rheumatic heart disease
Bone marrow transplant	Risk factors: irradiation of chest, age > 65, mucositis, acute graft-versus host disease
Infections	Bacterial or fungal pneumonia
Coagulopathy	Abnormal coagulation studies

Abbreviations: anti-GBM, anti-glomerular basement membrane; ANA, antinuclear antibodies; c-ANCA, cytoplasmic antineutrophil cytoplasmic antibodies; p-ANCA, perinuclear antineutrophil cytoplasmic antibodies.

10

possible vasculitis, but in many cases biopsy is necessary to confirm the diagnosis.

Bronchiolitis Obliterans-Organizing Pneumonia

Bronchiolitis obliterans-organizing pneumonia is characterized by the proliferation of granulation tissue in the respiratory bronchioles and alveolar ducts associated with chronic inflammation in the adjacent alveoli. BOOP may occur in association with a variety of other disorders, in which case it is a secondary form of BOOP. It may also occur in an isolated form, in which case it is idiopathic BOOP, also referred to as cryptogenic-organizing pneumonia. This discussion will focus on the idiopathic form of BOOP, emphasizing those points that help to distinguish it from other mimics of pneumonia.

Bronchiolitis obliterans-organizing pneumonia typically occurs in the fifth or sixth decade of life, with men and women being equally affected. The onset is typically subacute, with 75% of patients having symptoms less than 2 months in duration at the time of diagnosis. The typical presentation of BOOP begins with a flulike illness mimicking CAP, with fever, malaise, fatigue, dyspnea and dry cough. Rales are common, being present in approximately 75% of patients, but wheezes are rare as is clubbing. Laboratory tests are nonspecific, with the most common findings being an elevated sedimentation rate and leukocytosis.

The chest radiograph demonstrates bilateral, diffuse alveolar infiltrates, often with a peripheral distribution. Up to half of all patients will have recurrent or migratory infiltrates. Linear, interstitial and cavitary lesions are rare, as are pleural effusions and pleural thickening. CT scan typically reveals patchy, alveolar infiltrates with consolidation, ground-glass changes and bronchial-wall thickening.

The diagnosis of BOOP requires demonstration of the characteristic histologic pattern in the absence of other concurrent disease. Transbronchial biopsy is often insufficient to establish this diagnosis, since the histologic features of BOOP can be seen with a variety of other disorders. Therefore, open-lung biopsy remains the gold standard for diagnosing BOOP.

Eosinophilic Pneumonia Syndromes

The common pathologic feature of the eosinophilic pneumonia syndromes is the collection of eosinophils in the interstitial and alveolar spaces. Other pathologic findings that may be present to varying degrees include lymphocytic interstitial pneumonia, BOOP, and usual interstitial pneumonia. Only two diseases within this category are rapidly progressive and limited to the pulmonary system such that they are frequently mistaken for pneumonia. These are chronic eosinophilic pneumonia (CEP) and acute eosinophilic pneumonia.

Chronic Eosinophilic Pneumonia

Chronic eosinophilic pneumonia may often present as a fulminant illness with cough, fever, dyspnea, weight loss, wheezing, night sweats and radiographic infiltrates. With this constellation of findings, it is frequently mistaken for an infectious pneumonia.

Chronic eosinophilic pneumonia occurs most commonly in middle-aged adults, although it can occur at any age. Women are affected twice as often as men. Atopy is common, occurring in up to 50% of patients. Asthmatic symptoms occur in 30% to 50% of patients and are usually of recent onset. The onset is insidious and the course variable, with symptoms present for weeks prior to the time of diagnosis. Peripheral blood eosinophilia is present in more than 80% of patients and may be very high. Other nonspecific laboratory abnormalities include an elevated sedimentation rate, IgE levels, thrombocytosis, and iron deficiency anemia.

The chest radiograph demonstrates patchy, nonsegmental, alveolar infiltrates that tend to spare the central and basilar regions, resulting in a pattern termed the photographic negative of pulmonary edema. CT scan sometimes better delineates this peripheral pattern of disease, but the pattern is not pathognomonic and is not always present. However, this photonegative pulmonary edema pattern is so sufficiently rare that its presence should at least prompt consideration of the diagnosis of CEP. Other radiographic patterns that can be seen in CEP include diffuse bilateral infiltrates and lobar consolidation.

The diagnosis of CEP is usually suspected on clinical grounds based on the chest x-ray (CXR) pattern, blood eosinophilia and clinical history. However, examination of tissue is still necessary to confirm the diagnosis. The distinctive feature of CEP is elevated bronchoalveolar lavage (BAL) eosinophilia, typically in the 20% to 70% range. Transbronchial biopsy usually demonstrates interstitial and alveolar eosinophils and histiocytes. Multinucleated giant cells with a granulomatous component may be present as well. The sensitivity of BAL eosinophilia and transbronchial lung biopsy is such that open-lung biopsy is rarely needed to establish the diagnosis.

Fewer than 10% of patients will improve without treatment. Corticosteroids are the mainstay of therapy, with complete remission being the rule. Radiographic and clinical improvement can be expected within 2 to 3 days, with radiographic resolution by 3 weeks. Lack of a prompt response to corticosteroids should prompt reevaluation and consideration of other alternative diagnosis.

Although acute eosinophilic pneumonia (AEP) is characterized by eosinophilic infiltration of the lung parenchyma similar to that seen in CEP, the two syndromes seem to be distinct clinical entities.

Acute eosinophilic pneumonia occurs most commonly from the ages of 20 to 40, although it can occur at any age. Men are affected twice as often as women. There is no relationship to smoking, and unlike CEP, most patients do not have a history of asthma or atopy. In contrast to CEP, the onset of AEP is rapid, usually manifesting in less than 7 days. AEP typically presents with the onset of fever, nonproductive cough, dyspnea and pleuritic chest pain. Constitutional symptoms are common, including malaise, myalgia and night sweats. The most common findings on physical examination are fever, tachypnea, occasional rhonchi, and bibasilar crackles. Laboratory findings are similarly nonspecific. The peripheral eosinophil count usually becomes markedly elevated during the course of disease, but may be normal at presentation.

Early in AEP, the chest radiograph may only show subtle reticular or ground-glass infiltrates. High-resolution CT is more sensitive, demonstrating progressive, bilateral, patchy, ground-glass infiltrates, often located along the bronchovascular bundles. As the disease progresses, bilateral diffuse alveolar and reticular changes are seen. Unlike CEP, the infiltrates are not localized to the periphery. Small effusions occur in up to two thirds of patients and are frequently bilateral. If thoracentesis is done, these effusions typically demonstrate a high pH with marked eosinophilia.

The distinctive feature of AEP is the markedly elevated number of eosinophils in the BAL fluid. Typically greater than 25% of BAL cells are eosinophils, along with an increased proportion of BAL lymphocytes and neutrophils. Transbronchial biopsy usually demonstrates extensive eosinophilic parenchymal involvement, frequent diffuse alveolar damage, an organizing fibrinous exudate, hyaline membranes, type II cell hyperplasia and the absence of granulomas or hemorrhage.

Response to corticosteroids is frequently dramatic, occurring within 48 hours, and failure to respond should prompt the consideration of an alternative diagnosis. In contrast to CEP, there should be no further episodes of relapse during long-term follow-up.

Acute Interstitial Pneumonia

Acute interstitial pneumonia (AIP) is a rare, idiopathic form of diffuse alveolar damage. Hamman and Rich described AIP in 1935 and classified it with idiopathic pulmonary fibrosis. However, it is now recognized that AIP is separate and distinct from idiopathic pulmonary fibrosis and probably corresponds to a subset of idiopathic ARDS.

Acute interstitial pneumonia typically occurs in young healthy adults. There are no known risk factors and both sexes are affected equally. The median age is 43, with a range of 7 to 83 years of age. AIP typically presents after a prodromal period of up to 14 days with the abrupt onset of fever, cough and dyspnea. Chest radiographs usually demonstrate bilateral airspace disease. CT scan of the chest typically reveals patchy or diffuse areas of ground-glass attenuation. The disease is similar to ARDS, but unlike ARDS, there are none of the usual risk factors such as sepsis, shock, trauma or pneumonitis. Unlike idiopathic pulmonary fibrosis, the onset and progression of the disease is very rapid. Most patients develop hypoxic respiratory failure, and mechanical ventilation is often required. Mortality is high, ranging from 60% to 100% in several series, with an average of approximately 70%. It is unclear whether or not corticosteroids are beneficial in AIP, although most clinicians would favor a trial of corticosteroids once infectious etiologies have been ruled out. Thus AIP requires an open or thoracoscopic lung biopsy to confirm the diagnosis. The most common findings on biopsy are those of a proliferative picture of diffuse alveolar damage. Importantly, these features of diffuse alveolar damage are nonspecific and other diagnoses must be ruled out.

Pulmonary Alveolar Proteinosis

Pulmonary alveolar proteinosis (PAP), also known as pulmonary alveolar phospholipoproteinosis, is a rare diffuse lung disease characterized by the abnormal accumulation of lipoproteinaceous fluid in the distal airspaces. PAP probably represents a histopathologic syndrome caused by multiple etiologies. Histopathologic findings similar to PAP can be found in cases of silicoproteinosis, aluminum dust exposure, titanium exposure, hematologic malignancies, immunosuppressive disorders and opportunistic infections. However, despite these associations, the majority of cases of PAP are not associated with any of these risk factors and fall into the category of idiopathic PAP.

Pulmonary alveolar proteinosis typically presents with the insidious onset of dyspnea, fatigue, weight loss and low-grade fever. Most patients have a nonproductive cough, but occasionally a history of producing chunky or gelatinous material may be obtained. The age at presentation is usually 30 to 50 years, with men outnumbering women 2 to 1. Physical examination is remarkably normal in most patients, often with normal lung exams despite marked alveolar filling. Laboratory findings are nonspecific, with polycythemia, hypergammaglobulinemia and elevated lactate dehydrogenase being common.

Tests that can help differentiate PAP from other causes of nonresolving pneumonia include chest radiography, high-resolution CT, serum surfactant proteins, BAL fluid analysis and either open-lung biopsy or transbronchial biopsy. Chest radiographs typically demonstrate nonspecific central alveolar opacities in the lower- and mid-lung zones with marked sparing of the areas adjacent to the diaphragm and heart. High- resolution CT will often reveal a ground-glass appearance with thickening of the intralobular and interlobular septa in a pattern of polygonal shapes, frequently referred to as a "crazy paving" appearance. Elevated serum levels of surfactant proteins A and D have been demonstrated in PAP. These are not specific to PAP and can also be found in idiopathic pulmonary fibrosis. While none of these findings are diagnostic of PAP, they should raise the suspicion of PAP and can narrow the diagnostic possibilities.

Bronchoalveolar lavage, transbronchial biopsy or open biopsy can make the diagnosis. BAL demonstrates characteristic findings of PAP, including milky appearing, PAS-positive fluid, macrophages filled with PAS-positive material and acellular eosinophilic granules. Transbronchial biopsy is distinctive for preserved alveolar architecture with minimal thickening of the septa and scant inflammatory infiltrates. Terminal bronchioles and alveoli are flooded with a PAS-positive lipoproteinacious fluid consisting of phospholipids.

In contrast to many of the other noninfectious mimics of pneumonia, there is no role for immunosuppressives or corticosteroids in PAP. Indeed, PAP may exist with concurrent infections and predisposes to superinfections with *Nocardia*, opportunistic fungi, and mycobacteria. It is therefore critical to rule out concurrent infection, and corticosteroids should be avoided since there have been reports that they may increase mortality.

Sarcoidosis

Sarcoidosis is a chronic granulomatous disease of unknown etiology that affects multiple organ systems, most frequently the lungs, skin and eyes. Because sarcoidosis usually has extrapulmonary organ system involvement, it is rarely confused with other causes of nonresolving pneumonias. Evidence of extrapulmonary disease that should raise the suspicion of sarcoidosis includes extrathoracic lymphadenopathy, skin lesions such as erythema nodosum, lupus pernio or sarcoid plaques and uveitis. Clinically significant extrapulmonary involvement in other organ systems is much less common, with asymptomatic histologic evidence of involvement being the rule.

Chest radiographs typically demonstrate hilar adenopathy in more than 70% of cases, but parenchymal infiltrates in the absence of adenopathy may be present in up to 25% of cases. Histology typically demonstrates a nonspecific pattern of noncaseating granulomas with multinucleated giant cells and lymphocytes. In contrast to its use in many other interstitial lung diseases, bronchoscopy with transbronchial biopsy has an excellent diagnostic yield, in the range of 75% to 95%.

Since the finding of noncaseating granulomas is relatively nonspecific and may be found in other infectious and noninfectious granulomatous disorders, reserving therapy for those patients with severe or progressive disease is warranted. Therapy in such cases typically consists of corticosteroids given for several weeks to months.

■ Drug-Induced Pneumonitis

The number of drugs and therapeutic agents that may cause pulmonary toxicity is large and ever-growing. Mechanisms of injury include direct toxic effects, idiosyncratic reactions, and immune-mediated mechanisms. With some exceptions, the diagnosis of drug-

207

induced lung disease is one of exclusion. Clinical findings, histology, chest radiographs and even high-resolution CT scans are relatively nonspecific. Most reactions are not dose-related, but some reactions can occur weeks to years after the medication is discontinued. Thus to effectively rule out drug-induced lung disease in the setting of a nonresolving pneumonia requires careful evaluation of every drug that the patient is receiving or has recently received. A list of agents commonly associated with pulmonary toxicity that may mimic pneumonia is shown in Table 10.3. While it is impossible to review the almost limitless number of drugs with pulmonary toxicity, this section will focus on a few of the classic agents that have unusual or characteristic findings that may mimic pneumonia. These include amiodarone, methotrexate, and bleomycin.

Amiodarone

Amiodarone is associated with a wide variety of pulmonary presentations, including interstitial pneumonitis, mass lesions, BOOP, hypersensitivity pneumonitis, eosinophilic pneumonitis, diffuse alveolar hemorrhage, asthmalike syndromes, pleural effusions and lymphocytic interstitial pneumonitis. One unusual association of amiodarone toxicity is the possible association with postoperative ARDS. There are a number of reports of ARDS occurring after surgery in patients on amiodarone, typically within 18 to 72 hours. Some investigators have observed unilateral lung injury postoperatively, with only the ventilated lung being involved. Whether or not this represents potentiation of amiodarone toxicity by supplemental oxygen remains unclear.

The exact incidence of these complications is difficult to define, with most estimates being around 5% in the literature. There are no good ways to identify those patients at particularly high risk for amiodarone toxicity. Men are affected more commonly than women, and pulmonary toxicity is more common in those with other pulmonary comorbidities. Most patients who develop toxicity are on 400 mg per day or more for 2 or more months. As with most forms of drug toxicity, clinical and radiographic findings are otherwise nonspecific. Symptoms may be acute or insidious in onset. Pleurisy is uncommon, occurring in 10% of cases, with pleural effusions also being uncommon but reported. Chest radiograph is nonspecific, ranging from focal alveolar infiltrates to peripheral infiltrates to mixed alveolar-interstitial patterns. Because amiodarone is an iodinated compound, its density on noncontrast high-resolution CT scan may be increased. While not sensitive, this is one of the few highly specific radiographic findings that, when present, can definitively establish a diagnosis.

Treatment for suspected amiodarone toxicity is corticosteroids and discontinuation of the drug. In those rare instances when there are no suitable alternative antiarrhythmic agents, corticosteroids combined with reducing amiodarone to the lowest possible dose may be effective.

Methotrexate

Methotrexate has been associated with many syndromes that may mimic pneumonia, including bronchospasm, BOOP, pleural effusions, eosinophilic pulmonary infiltrates, noncardiogenic pulmonary edema (from intrathecal methotrexate) and a hypersensitivity type of pneumonitis. Because opportunistic infection is a well-documented complication with even low-dose methotrexate, it is particularly important to rule out concurrent infection and to look for signs that may differentiate drug toxicity from infection. In patients receiving chemotherapeutic doses of methotrexate, there are well-described cases of a hypersensitivity pneumonitislike reaction, with about half of patients reporting both lung and blood eosinophilia. Granulomas are also frequently associated with this reaction, and occasionally hilar adenopathy has been reported.

Patients receiving lower doses of methotrexate for anti-inflammatory purposes have a slightly different presentation. About 5% of patients receiving chronic low dose of methotrexate develop a subacute interstitial process with fever, hypoxia, rales and cough. Eosinophilia in this syndrome is rare, but poorly formed granulomas are still seen on biopsy. Nitrofurantoin potentiates this syndrome, and deaths have been reported. Treatment is drug withdrawal and corticosteroids.

Bleomycin

Bleomycin has been associated with a wide variety of complications, including pulmonary fibrosis, BOOP, eosinophilic infiltrates, pulmonary veno-occlusive disease and an acute pneumonitis reaction similar to hypersensitivity. Up to 20% of patients on bleomycin develop pulmonary reactions, and 1% die of pulmonary complications. Risk factors include age above 70 years and dose greater than 450 u. There is a marked synergy between bleomycin and high levels of inspired oxygen. This is often encountered after general anesthesia, typically manifesting about 18 hours later as ARDS. Other reported synergistic insults include the concurrent use of granulocyte colony-stimulating factor. Treatment in all cases includes minimizing inspired oxygen content and corticosteroids.

■ Pulmonary Vascular Disease

Vascular conditions that may mimic pneumonia include pulmonary embolism (PE) and congestive heart failure. PE is a common problem with radiographic and clinical findings that may easily be mistaken for pneumonia. There are no specific or typical clinical signs and symptoms. Dyspnea is observed in 80% of patients, pleuritic pain in up to 75%, hemoptysis in 20% and wheezing in 15%. Chest radiographs show infiltrates in up to 30% of cases, with effusions being present in 20%. Other radiographic findings include diaphragmatic elevation in 60%, focal oligemia in 10%, enlarged pulmonary arteries in 20% and normal radiographs in 30%. The classic "Hampton's Hump" is rarely seen. Infiltrates from PE may take several weeks to resolve and thus are easily mistaken for slowly resolving pneumonia.

Although the chest radiograph does not correlate with the severity of PE, the alveolar-arterial gradient on blood gas correlates linearly with the severity of PE. The possibility of PE as the cause of a non-resolving pneumonia syndrome should be raised when hypoxia is out of proportion to radiographic findings and fails to improve.

Although the diagnosis of congestive heart failure is usually apparent, occasionally unusual radiographic patterns of cardiogenic pulmonary edema may mimic pneumonia. In particular, atypical pulmonary edema patterns have been well described in patients with bullous lung disease and in patients with mitral regurgitation. Because pulmonary edema principally develops in areas of maximal perfusion, patients with marked COPD may manifest asymmetric pulmonary edema patterns. Similarly, if the regurgitant jet associated with mitral valve insufficiency is directed at one of the pulmonary veins, unilateral and focal pulmonary edema patterns may occur. In this setting, echocardiography may be of help to identify the severity and direction of the mitral regurgitation. In borderline cases, Swan-Ganz catheterization may be necessary to further clarify the issue and is usually definitive.

SUGGESTED READING

Afessa B, Greaves WL, Frederick WR. Pneumococcal bacteremia in adults: a 14-year experience in an inner-city university hospital. *Clin Infect Dis*. 1995;21:345-351.

Allen JN, Pacht ER, Gadek JE, Davis WB. Acute eosinophilic pneumonia as a reversible cause of noninfectious respiratory failure. *N Engl J Med*. 1989;321:569-574.

Allen JN, Davis WB. Eosinophilic lung diseases. *Am J Respir Crit Care Med*. 1994;150(pt 1):1423-1438.

American Thoracic Society. Hospital-acquired pneumonia in adults: diagnosis, assessment of severity, initial antimicrobial therapy, and preventive strategies. A consensus statement. *Am J Respir Crit Care Med*. 1996;153:1711-1725.

Ampel NM, Dols CL, Galgiani JN. Coccidioidomycosis during human immunodeficiency virus infection: results of a prospective study in a coccidioidal endemic area. *Am J Med*. 1993;94:235-240.

Appropriate uses of human immunoglobulin in clinical practice: memorandum from an IUIS/WHO meeting. *Bull World Health Organ*. 1982;60:43-47.

Baselski VS, Wunderink RG. Bronchoscopic diagnosis of pneumonia. *Clin Microbiol Rev*. 1994;7:533-558.

Bass JB Jr, Farer LS, Hopewell PC, et al. Treatment of tuberculosis and tuberculosis infection in adults and children. American Thoracic Society and The Centers for Disease Control and Prevention. *Am J Respir Crit Care Med*. 1994;149:1359-1374.

Berkman N, Breuer R. Pulmonary involvement in lymphoma. *Respir Med*. 1993;87:85-92.

Binder RE, Faling LJ, Pugatch RD, Mahasaen C, Snider GL. Chronic necrotizing pulmonary aspergillosis: a discrete clinical entity. *Medicine*. 1982;61:109-124.

Buckley RH, Schiff RI. The use of intravenous immune globulin in immunodeficiency diseases. *N Engl J Med*. 1991;325:110-117.

Buschman DL, Waldron JA Jr, King TE Jr. Churg-Strauss pulmonary vasculitis. High-resolution computed tomography scanning and pathologic findings. *Am Rev Respir Dis*. 1990;142:458-461.

Chin DP, Yajko DM, Hadley WK, et al. Clinical utility of a commercial test based on the polymerase chain reaction for detecting *Mycobacterium* tuberculosis in respiratory specimens. *Am J Respir Crit Care Med*. 1995;151:1872-1877.

Coblentz C. The chest radiograph in the acquired immunodeficieny syndrome. *Semin Resp Med*. 1992;13:275-292.

Cordier JF. Cryptogenic organizing pneumonitis. Bronchiolitis obliterans organizing pneumonia. *Clin Chest Med*. 1993;14:677-692.

Counsell SR, Tan JS, Dittus RS. Unsuspected pulmonary tuberculosis in a community teaching hospital. *Arch Intern Med*. 1989; 149:1274-1278.

Davies SF, Sarosi GA. Role of serodiagnostic tests and skin tests in the diagnosis of fungal disease. *Clin Chest Med*. 1987;8:135-146.

Denning DW, Follansbee SE, Scolaro M, Norris S, Edelstein H, Stevens DA. Pulmonary aspergillosis in the acquired immunodeficiency syndrome. *N Engl J Med*. 1991;324:654-662.

Dumont P, Gasser B, Rougé C, Massard G, Wihlm JM. Bronchoalveolar carcinoma: histopathologic study of evolution in a series of 105 surgically treated patients. *Chest*. 1998;113:391-395.

Duna GF, Galperin C, Hoffman GS. Wegener's granulomatosis. *Rheum Dis Clin North Am*. 1995;21:949-986.

Ebara H, Ikezoe J, Johkok T, et al. Chronic eosinophilic pneumonia: evolution of chest radiograms and CT features. *J Comput Assist Tomogr*. 1994;18:737-744.

Ellner PD, Kiehn TE, Cammarata R, Hosmer M. Rapid detection and identification of pathogenic mycobacteria by combining radiometric and nucleic acid probe methods. *J Clin Micobiol*. 1988;26:1349-1352.

Goodwin RA, Loyd JE, Des Prez RM. Histoplasmosis in normal hosts. *Medicine*. 1981;60:231-266.

Gordon JD, MacKeen AD, Marrie TJ, Fraser DB. The radiographic features of epidemic and sporadic Q fever pneumonia. *J Can Assoc Radiol*. 1984;35:293-296.

Grossman CB, Bragg DG, Armstrong D. Roentgen manifestations of pulmonary nocardiosis. *Radiology*. 1970;96:325-330.

Harber P, Terry PB. Fatal lung abscesses: review of 11 years' experience. *South Med J*. 1981;74:281-283.

Hoffman GS, Kerr GS, Leavitt RY, et al. Wegener granulomatosis: an analysis of 158 patients. *Ann Intern Med*. 1992;116:488-498.

Hofmann J, Cetron MS, Farley MM, et al. The prevalence of drug-resistant *Streptococcus pneumoniae* in Atlanta. *N Engl J Med*. 1995;333:481-486.

Hunninghake GW, Gilbert S, Pueringer R, et al. Outcome of the treatment for sarcoidosis. *Am J Respir Crit Care Med*. 1994;149(pt 1):893-898.

Jacobs MR. Treatment and diagnosis of infections caused by drug-resistant *Streptococcus pneumoniae*. *Clin Infect Dis*. 1992;15:119-127.

Jederlinic PJ, Sicilian L, Gaensler EA. Chronic eosinophilic pneumonia. A report of 19 cases and a review of the literature. *Medicine*. 1988;67:154-162.

Katzenstein AL, Myers JL, Mazur MT. Acute interstitial pneumonia. A clinicopathologic, ultrastructural, and cell kinetic study. *Am J Surg Pathol*. 1986;10:256-267.

Kemper CA, Hostetler JS, Follansbee SE, et al. Ulcerative and plaque-like tracheobronchitis due to infection with *Aspergillus* in patients with AIDS. *Clin Infect Dis*. 1993;17:344.

Kovacs JA, Hiemenz JW, Macher AM, et al. *Pneumocystis carinii* pneumonia: a comparison between patients with the acquired immunodeficiency syndrome and patients with other immunodeficiencies. *Ann Intern Med*. 1984;100:663-671.

Leatherman JW. The lung in systemic vasculitis. *Semin Respir Infect*. 1988;3:274-288.

Ludington LG, Verska JJ, Howard T, Kypridakis G, Brewer LA III. Bronchiolar carcinoma (alveolar cell), another great imitator; a review of 41 cases. *Chest*. 1972;61:622-628.

Mark EJ, Ramirez JF. Pulmonary capillaritis and hemorrhage in patients with systemic vasculitis. *Arch Pathol Lab Med*. 1985;109:413.

Miller WT Jr, Sais GJ, Frank I, Gefter WB, Aronchick JM, Miller WT. Pulmonary aspergillosis in patients with AIDS. Clinical and radiographic correlations. *Chest*. 1994;105:37-44.

Moreno F, Crisp C, Jorgensen JH, Patterson JE. The clinical and molecular epidemiology of bacteremias at a university hospital caused by pneumococci not susceptible to penicillin. *J Infect Dis.* 1995;172:427-432.

Naughton M, Fahy J, FitzGerald MX. Chronic eosinophilic pneumonia. A long-term follow-up of 12 patients. *Chest.* 1993;103:162-165.

Olson J, Colby TV, Elliott CG. Hamman-Rich syndrome revisited. *Mayo Clin Proc.* 1990;65:1538-1548.

Primack SL, Hartman TE, Ikezoe J, et al. Acute interstitial pneumonia: radiographic and CT findings in nine patients. *Radiology.* 1993;188:817.

Pallares R, Liñares J, Vadillo M, et al. Resistance to penicillin and cephalosporin and mortality from severe pneumococcal pneumonia in Barcelona, Spain [published erratum appears in *N Engl J Med.* 1995;333:1655]. *N Engl J Med.* 1995;333:474-480.

Pallares R, Gudiol F, Liñares J, et al. Risk factors and response to antibiotic therapy in adults with bacteremic pneumonia caused by penicillin-resistant pneumococci. *N Engl J Med.* 1987;317:18-22.

PIOPED Investigators. Value of the ventilation/perfusion scan in acute pulmonary embolism. Results of the prospective investigation of pulmonary embolism diagnosis (PIOPED). *JAMA.* 1990; 263:2753-2759.

Pope-Harman AL, Davis WB, Allen ED, Christoforidis AJ, Allen JN. Acute eosinophilic pneumonia. A summary of 15 cases and review of the literature. *Medicine.* 1996;75:334-342.

Prakash UB, Barham SS, Carpenter HA, Dines DE, Marsh HM. Pulmonary alveolar phospolipoproteinosis: experience with 34 cases and a review. *Mayo Clin Proc.* 1987;62:499-518.

Rao JK, Weinberger M, Oddone EZ, Allen NB, Landsman P, Feussner JR. The role of antineutrophil cytoplasmic antibody (c-ANCA) testing in the diagnosis of Wegener granulomatosis. A literature review and meta-analysis. *Ann Intern Med.* 1995;123:925-932.

Rodrigues J, Niederman MS, Fein AM, Pai PB. Nonresolving pneumonia in steroid-treated patients with obstructive lung disease. *Am J Med.* 1992;93:29-34.

215

Rosenow EC III, Myers JL, Swensen SJ, Pisani RJ. Drug-induced pulmonary disease. An update. *Chest*. 1992;102:239-250.

Sarosi GA, Johnson PC. Disseminated histoplasmosis in patients infected with human immunodeficiency virus. *Clin Infect Dis*. 1992;14(suppl 1):S60-S67.

Sawyer LA, Fishbein DB, McDade JE. Q fever: current concepts. *Rev Infect Dis*. 1987;9:935-946.

Screening for tuberculosis and tuberculous infection in high-risk populations. Recommendations of the Advisory Committe for Elimination of Tuberculosis. *Morb Mortal Wkly Rep*. 1990;39:1-7.

Skull S, Kemp A. Treatment of hypogammaglobulinaemia with intravenous immunoglobulin, 1973-93. *Arch Dis Child*. 1996;74:527-530.

Sosenko A, Glassroth J. Fiberoptic bronchoscopy in the evaluation of lung abscesses. *Chest*. 1985;87:489-494.

Thomas PD, Hunninghake GW. Current concepts of the pathogenesis of sarcoidosis. *Am Rev Respir Dis*. 1987;135:747-760.

Tobler A, Schürch E, Altermatt HJ, Im Hof V. Anti-basement membrane antibody disease with severe pulmonary hemorrhage and normal renal function. *Thorax*. 1991;46:68-70.

Travis WD, Colby TV, Lombard C, Carpenter HA. A clinicopathologic study of 34 cases of diffuse pulmonary hemorrhage with lung biopsy confirmation. *Am J Surg Pathol*. 1990;14:1112-1125.

Umeki S, Soejima R. Acute and chronic eosinophilic pneumonia: clinical evaluation and the criteria. *Intern Med*. 1992;31:847-856.

Update: tuberculosis elimination–United States. *Morb Mortal Wkly Rep*. 1990;39:153-156.

Yoshida K, Shijubo N, Koba H, et al. Chronic eosinophilic pneumonia progressing to lung fibrosis. *Eur Respir J*. 1994;7:1541-1544.

Zitnik RJ, Cooper JA Jr. Pulmonary disease due to antirheumatic agents. *Clin Chest Med*. 1990;11:139-150.

11 Approach to Nonresolving Pneumonia

In developing a diagnostic approach, it is important to first understand the capabilities as well as the limitations of the most commonly employed diagnostic tests. Careful consideration of the diagnostic yield, risks and benefits is critical in deciding whether additional invasive tests are warranted (Figure 11.1). The diagnostic tests that are most commonly employed in evaluating nonresolving pneumonia are:

- Chest radiographs
- Chest computed tomography (CT) scans
- Fiberoptic bronchoscopy
- Open-lung biopsy.

Radiographic Tools

As is clear from Chapter 9, *Natural History of Pneumonia*, and Chapter 10, *Possible Etiologies of Nonresolving Pneumonia*, radiographic findings alone are almost never specific for any one diagnosis. However, radiographic studies are useful in narrowing the differential diagnosis and suggesting groups of diagnostic possibilities for consideration. The primary radiographic tools in assessing nonresolving pneumonia are chest radiographs and chest CT scans. The evaluation of nonresolving pneumonia has further benefited from the development of high-resolution chest CT (HRCT). HRCT involves using thin-section scanning at 1 to 2 mm collimation combined with a high spatial reconstruction algorithm. HRCT is superior to conventional techniques in several key ar-

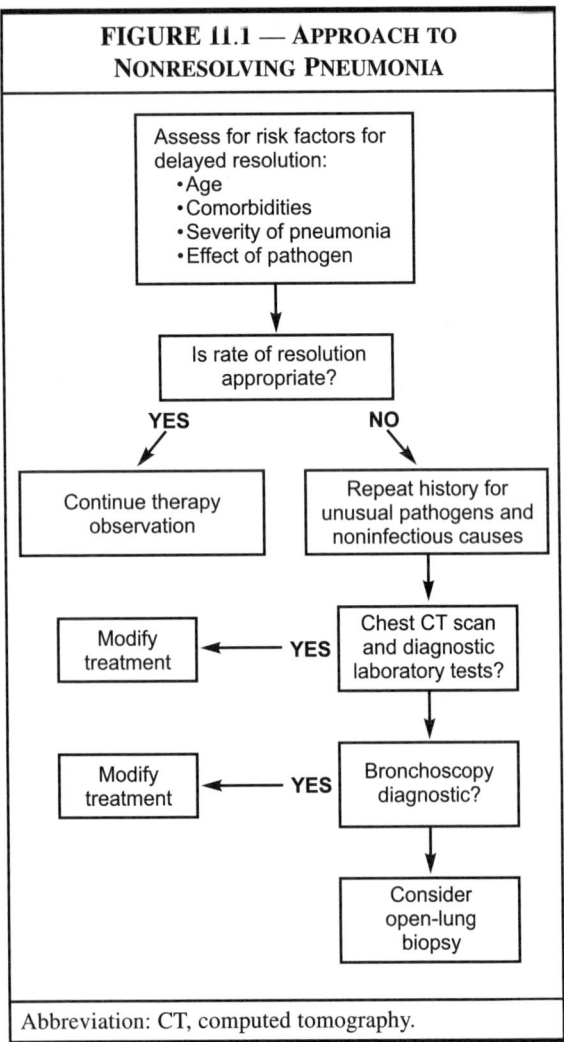

FIGURE 11.1 — APPROACH TO NONRESOLVING PNEUMONIA

Assess for risk factors for delayed resolution:
- Age
- Comorbidities
- Severity of pneumonia
- Effect of pathogen

↓

Is rate of resolution appropriate?

YES → Continue therapy observation

NO → Repeat history for unusual pathogens and noninfectious causes

↓

Chest CT scan and diagnostic laboratory tests?

YES → Modify treatment

↓

Bronchoscopy diagnostic?

YES → Modify treatment

↓

Consider open-lung biopsy

Abbreviation: CT, computed tomography.

eas that impact on the management of nonresolving pneumonia. Compared with conventional chest x-ray, HRCT allows superior detection of parenchymal abnormalities, including emphysema, airspace disease, interstitial disease and nodules. Detection of these structural abnormalities may narrow the differential diagnosis or suggest new possibilities.

Certain conditions, such as amiodarone toxicity and lymphangitic spread of malignancy have specific HRCT characteristics that may suggest a diagnosis with reasonable specificity. In addition, the greater sensitivity of HRCT allows for better precision in assessing a patient's response to therapy over time. This is especially useful when there is preexisting lung disease that makes it difficult to distinguish acute from chronic changes. CT also improves detection of localized collections, such as abscesses and empyema. Finally, the ability to better localize disease helps direct biopsy procedures and may improve diagnostic yield.

Bronchoscopy

The role of fiberoptic bronchoscopy (FOB) in the diagnosis of nonresolving pneumonia depends largely on the clinical scenario. The best accepted indication for FOB in the diagnosis of pneumonia is in the immunocompromised host with diffuse pulmonary infiltrates. In this setting, different organisms that require markedly different treatments may have similar or indistinguishable clinical presentations. While clinical and radiographic patterns may narrow the set of diagnostic possibilities, abnormal host factors, poor baseline cardiopulmonary reserve and the wide spectrum of possible pathogens often make an empiric trial risky and therefore justify early FOB. Similarly, in cases of nonresolving pneumonia, the relative ease and low risk of FOB make this an appealing diagnostic procedure in a population of patients with a similarly wide spectrum of possible infectious and noninfectious etiologies.

Despite the frequency of its use for this indication, there are few studies that document the diagnostic yield of FOB for nonresolving pneumonia. Retrospective analysis of FOB for nonresolving pneumonia demonstrates that FOB is used successfully to diagnose 86% to 95% of patients who eventually have a specific diagnosis established. FOB is more likely to establish a specific diagnosis in younger, nonsmoking patients with multilobar involvement and prolonged duration of disease. Patients older than 55 years of age, smokers and those with immune defects are more likely to have a nondiagnostic bronchoscopy and to have slowly resolving pneumonia.

The utility of FOB in nonresolving pneumonia also depends upon the disease possibilities being considered and the population being studied. FOB will be most useful in diagnosing unusual pathogens, some immunologic disorders such as chronic and acute eosinophilic pneumonia and neoplastic diseases. Again, depending upon the diseases being considered, transbronchial biopsy may or may not be necessary. In other situations, FOB may have a relatively low diagnostic yield but may provide useful information in ruling out infectious processes. This is especially important if immunosuppressive therapy is being considered.

The role of bronchoscopy in ruling out bacterial infections in the setting of nonresolving pneumonia is unclear. Most recommendations are based upon extrapolating data from studies of community-acquired pneumonia (CAP) and nosocomial pneumonia. Since the causative organism in CAP is not isolated in more than 40% of cases, the initial role of

FOB is limited. FOB for CAP, particularly if done prior to antibiotic therapy, increases the percentage of cases with a defined etiology. However, the additional pathogens that are isolated are almost always covered by routine empiric antibiotic therapy. Therefore, the role of FOB in identifying bacterial pathogens in non-resolving CAP is not easily defined. Unless unusual pathogens such as tuberculosis are present, the diagnostic sensitivity and specificity for pathogens in this population is probably limited.

Based upon studies of ventilator-associated pneumonia (VAP), however, several recommendations can be made. First, unprotected collection techniques, such as tracheal aspirates and unprotected bronchoalveolar lavage, are of little value for bacterial pathogens. While multiple protected bronchoscopic techniques have been utilized, each with their own particular advantages and disadvantages, it is unclear if any one technique is markedly superior. Techniques include protected specimen brush and protected bronchoalveolar lavage with quantitative culture.

The important point with all of these techniques is to obtain specimens from the distal alveolar or respiratory bronchiole with minimal proximal airway contamination. Controversy persists whether diagnostic bronchoscopy should be performed on all patients with VAP since multiple studies have shown no survival benefit compared with that achieved with empiric therapy alone. Whether or not this applies to nonresolving pneumonia is unclear. Certainly FOB that detects noninfectious etiologies would be expected to alter therapy and presumably impact on survival. Given these limited data, it is still best to utilize a protected specimen technique if bacterial pathogens are suspected, realizing the limitations of the technique.

Open-Lung Biopsy

While definitive recommendations on the decision
to proceed to open-lung biopsy cannot be made, several factors need to be considered when deciding on
whether to proceed with open-lung biopsy. These factors include disease progression, the diagnostic possibilities being considered and the effect that a positive open-lung biopsy will have on treatment. In general, if the disease is relatively stable, a period of careful observation may be warranted. If there is a high
likelihood for a disease that would necessitate a dramatic change in therapy, open-lung biopsy is warranted. Diseases in this category generally include
most vasculitis syndromes (Wegener's) and inflammatory lung diseases that require immunosuppression. In
these cases, the risk of immunosuppression in a patient who is currently infected requires a specific tissue diagnosis. The more potent the immunosuppression required, the more open-lung biopsy is warranted.
Similarly, FOB in these cases can help to rule out concurrent infection, but open-lung biopsy to establish the
diagnosis remains the gold standard.

Summary

The diagnostic evaluation of nonresolving pneumonia begins with a careful history, physical examination and review of the medical record. The goal is
to determine whether or not the rate of resolution is
within the range of expected norms, taking into consideration the patient's underlying host factors,
comorbidities, severity of illness and any known
pathogens. If the patient is stable or slowly improving and has other comorbidities or host factors which
are known to delay the rate of resolution of pneumonia, careful observation and continued therapy are

warranted for 4 to 8 weeks. If there is no resolution or progression of disease, a more aggressive diagnostic approach is warranted.

The physician must first determine whether the nonresolving pneumonia is due to an infectious or a noninfectious etiology. The initial evaluation should include a chest CT scan to look for unsuspected nodules or localized collections of fluid. Any significant pleural collections should be biopsied or drained. If this is unrevealing, bronchoscopy should be considered.

Several factors should be considered when deciding on whether to proceed with FOB. As mentioned earlier, in cases with stable but nonresolving pneumonia with impaired host defenses, it is reasonable to observe the patient, since the infection can be expected to take a longer time to clear. When infection fails to resolve in a patient without impaired host defenses or if there is clinical progression, FOB should be pursued. Similarly, if noninfectious etiologies or unusual pathogens are suspected, FOB is warranted. Positive results from FOB can serve to modify or optimize treatment regimens.

Similarly, a negative result has significant value. Patients with a negative FOB have a good chance of merely having a slowly resolving pneumonia and if they are stable can be observed. Similarly, a negative FOB will narrow the differential diagnosis in patients with progressive disease. Diseases that typically are not diagnosed with FOB that are progressive include pulmonary vasculitis syndromes, bronchiolitis obliterans-organizing pneumonia, and the various forms of diffuse alveolar damage. In these cases, a negative bronchoscopy with progressive symptoms should prompt consideration of an open-lung biopsy.

12 Parapneumonic Effusions and Empyema

Pleural effusions complicate up to 40% of bacterial pneumonias. They vary in severity, ranging from uncomplicated effusions to empyema. Some require only antibiotics and observation, while others require chest tube drainage or even surgery. Thus, treatment of parapneumonic effusions requires knowledge of:
- Pathogenesis of parapneumonic effusions
- Appropriate imaging
- Pleural fluid analysis
- Assessment of the risk for complications
- Choosing appropriate interventions.

Pathogenesis

Parapneumonic effusions can be divided into three stages:
- Uncomplicated parapneumonic effusions
- Complicated parapneumonic effusions
- Empyema.

Although classified as distinct stages, it is important to realize that these stages actually represent a continuum of disease rather than rigid classes. The importance of understanding these stages lies in the prognostic value that each stage is associated with and thus the treatment implications that go with each stage.

■ Uncomplicated Parapneumonic Effusion

The first stage is that of uncomplicated parapneumonic effusion. In this stage, an exudative effusion forms during the first 72 hours when the resorptive capacity of the pleural space is exceeded. These effusions are usually predominantly neutrophilic in nature, typically with total neutrophil counts in excess of 10,000/mL, and will usually resolve with resolution of the pneumonia. Because of this, they do not require chest tube drainage or other invasive measures.

■ Complicated Parapneumonic Effusions

Some uncomplicated parapneumonic effusions will progress to become complicated effusions. This may occur if there is persistent bacterial contamination of the pleural space. With persistent infection, there is an increase in the number of neutrophils in the pleural space as well as a corresponding pleural fluid acidosis. This acidosis is characterized by a pleural fluid pH in the range of 7.1 to 7.3 and is caused by anaerobic glucose metabolism by both neutrophils and bacteria.

As neutrophils persist and subsequently lyse within the pleural space, the pleural fluid lactate dehydrogenase (LDH) increases, often in excess of 1000 IU/L. Persistent inflammation leads to deposition of a dense layer of fibrin on both the visceral and parietal pleura that may subsequently lead to loculations and adhesions. Importantly, cultures of the pleural fluid at this point may be sterile, since bacteria can be cleared relatively rapidly while still initiating this fibrinopurulent stage. The fibrinopurulent stage may last anywhere from 3 to 7 days.

■ Empyema

In the third stage, empyema develops, with the accumulation of pus within the pleural space. Bacteria may be evident on Gram stain of the pleural fluid. A positive culture or Gram stain is not always present, however, since patients may be infected with anaerobic organisms that are difficult to isolate. Similarly, patients may have been on antibiotics prior to pleural fluid collection, significantly lowering the diagnostic yield of subsequent cultures.

Finally, many times empyema will be loculated and the pleural fluid aspirate may represent only a sterile inflammatory area adjacent to an infected loculation (Figure 12.1). As the infection persists, additional neutrophils are recruited, resulting in even more severe pleural fluid acidosis as well as a marked decrease in pleural fluid glucose. Eventually, a thick pleural peel develops, encasing and entrapping the lung as it organizes. This organizational phase of empyema usually occurs over 2 to 3 weeks. Importantly, not all organisms are equally likely to cause empyema. The most common organisms causing empyema are shown in Table 12.1.

Imaging of Pleural Effusions

Initial imaging of pleural effusions is usually accomplished with a plain chest radiograph. Other adjunctive measures include computed tomography (CT) of the chest and ultrasound. These are usually reserved for more difficult cases when there may be a question of loculations, concurrent chest masses or to help guide thoracentesis. The basic chest radiograph remains the best initial choice and can provide substantial information rapidly.

On a plain upright posterior-anterior and lateral chest film, up to 75 mL of effusion can occupy the subpulmonic space without spillover. As the amount of fluid increases above 75 mL the lateral chest radiograph demonstrates obliteration of the posterior costophrenic sulcus. Once a minimum of 175 mL is present the lateral costophrenic angle is obscured as well. At 1000 mL, the effusion will typically reach approximately the fourth intercostal space anteriorly.

Decubitus radiographs with the patient in both lateral decubitus positions are useful to further evalu-

FIGURE 12.1 — EMPYEMA

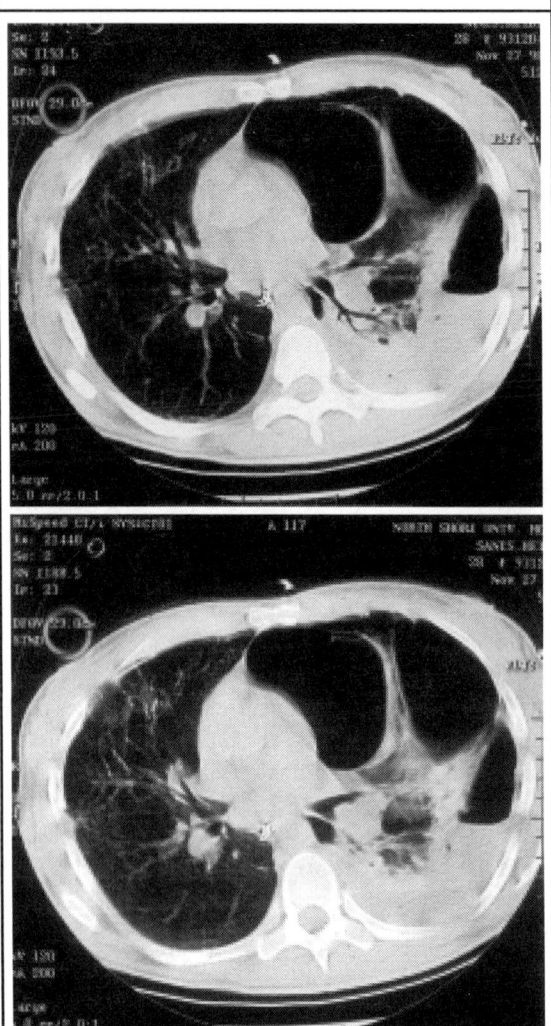

Chest radiograph and computed tomography (CT) scan demonstrating a loculated empyema secondary to pneumococcal pneumonia with septic shock.

TABLE 12.1 — CAUSES OF EMPYEMA	
Organism	**Percent**
Anaerobes	30 to 70
Staphylococcus aureus	25 to 35
Gram-negative bacilli	20 to 30
Streptococcus pneumoniae	5 to 15
Culture negative	3 to 30
Polymicrobial	30 to 70

ate the effusion. Free-flowing effusions that are thicker than 10 mm on a lateral decubitus film are usually amenable to thoracentesis. For quantification purposes:

- Small effusions usually will be less than 15 mm thick on decubitus view.
- Moderate effusions will be 15 to 45 mm thick.
- Large effusions will be greater than 45 mm thick.

While a plain chest radiograph is the primary tool for the initial evaluation of effusions it does have several important limitations, primarily related to patient positioning, subpulmonic effusions and loculated effusions. Mobile effusions may layer along the posterior chest in supine patients, leading to underestimation of the amount of pleural fluid. As the effusion layers along the posterior thorax, it produces a diffuse veil-like effect throughout the entire chest that may be missed or interpreted as airspace disease. This will appear as a diffuse haziness throughout all lung fields. Distinguishing this from parenchymal lung disease may be difficult. Features that suggest a posterior effusion rather than parenchymal disease include the absence of air bronchograms and visible pulmonary vessels throughout the area of increased opacity created by the effusion.

Subpulmonic effusions may elevate the lung bases while producing minimal costophrenic-angle blunting. If the fluid is free flowing, a lateral decubitus film will serve to readily identify this problem. Features that suggest a subpulmonic effusion include shifting of the apex of the diaphragm laterally, diaphragmatic inversion, making the diaphragm appear concave and separation of the lung from the stomach bubble greater than 2 cm.

Loculated effusions are the result of adhesions. Adhesions may arise from preexisting disease or may be a consequence of the pneumonia itself. Because the fluid is not free flowing, loculated effusions will not necessarily layer on lateral decubitus films and may be mistaken for parenchymal masses or consolidation. Loculation is frequently encountered when hemothorax, empyema, chylothorax and tuberculous infection cause the effusion. Features that suggest a loculated effusion include an obtuse angle between the pleural mass and the chest wall, a smooth border and homogenous density.

While specific features may help to identify some subpulmonic and loculated effusions, in many cases these findings may be absent or not specific enough to allow an accurate assessment. In these cases, additional imaging with either CT or ultrasound may be useful.

Computed tomography has several advantages over routine chest radiographs. Chest CT has increased sensitivity for small effusions when compared with regular chest radiographs. As little as 2 to 10 mL of pleural fluid can be detected on chest CT. In supine patients and in those with subpulmonic effusions, fluid is easily visualized, even in the posterior and subpulmonic locations. In those with loculated effusions or underlying parenchymal processes, CT allows visualization and differentiation of the underlying parenchyma from the pleural effusion. CT also images the pleura more accurately, allowing more precise measurement of pleural thickness.

Finally, CT may help to distinguish empyema from lung abscess. In the fibrinopurulent and organizing stages of empyema, CT will demonstrate strong enhancement of the visceral and parietal pleurae, producing the so-called split pleura sign. In addition, with empyema formation, there is usually concurrent thickening of the pleura during the fibrinopurulent and organizing phases that may only be apparent on CT.

Ultrasonography is the other imaging modality commonly employed to evaluate pleural effusions. Ultrasound easily identifies free or loculated effusions and facilitates differentiation of loculated effusions from any underlying mass. This is especially useful in guiding thoracentesis procedures. With ultrasound guidance, effusions that would normally be too small to undergo thoracentesis can be drained. Loculated effusions are also easier to drain under ultrasound guidance, allowing the clinician to identify and drain the largest collections within any given effusion. Thus ultrasound-guided thoracentesis is a relatively quick and easy technique to collect pleural fluid for diagnostic assessment. However, CT remains the method of choice for more complicated interventions, such as catheter placement for empyema drainage or biopsy of pleural lesions.

Pleural Fluid Analysis

In the setting of a pleural effusion of unknown cause, pleural fluid analysis is critical to rapidly identifying a specific etiology. Pleural fluid analysis in combination with clinical judgment allows an accurate diagnosis in 75% of patients. Even when nondiagnostic, pleural fluid analysis can be useful in excluding certain diagnosis. Thus clinical decision making is influenced by pleural fluid analysis in over 90% of cases. While observation of a pleural effusion may be warranted in other clinical settings, such as when there is congestive heart failure, in the setting of pneumonia, early thoracentesis is usually warranted to rule out empyema and to obtain cultures to help guide antibiotic therapy. Therefore, early thoracentesis to obtain pleural fluid for analysis should be attempted whenever there is more than 10 mm of fluid on lateral decubitus films. In those patients with smaller effusions, ultrasound guidance may be utilized to aid in obtaining pleural fluid samples. In cases where the effusion is too small for even ultrasound-guided thoracentesis, serial chest radiographs should be obtained to confirm that the effusion has not progressed while the patient has been undergoing treatment.

Initial fluid analysis should include observation of the gross appearance of the fluid, Gram stain, culture, pleural fluid LDH, protein, glucose, pH, cell count, and differential. Other tests that may be useful include pleural fluid amylase, triglycerides, cholesterol and adenosine deaminase. Table 12.2 summarizes the conditions associated with each of these tests.

Parapneumonic effusions are usually exudative in nature. If thoracentesis of a pleural effusion indicates a transudative effusion in the setting of clinical pneumonia, this should lead to consideration of other concurrent diseases that may cause a transudative effusion, such as congestive heart failure. In patients with bilateral effusions, one side may rarely demonstrate a transudative pattern while the other side demonstrates an exudative pattern.

Bacterial parapneumonic effusions are typically neutrophilic exudative effusions. Lymphocytic exudative effusions are characteristic of tuberculous pleural effusions as well as malignant effusions. In the

TABLE 12.2 — PLEURAL FLUID ANALYSIS	
Test	**Condition**
Gram stain	Positive Gram stain suggests empyema
Lactate dehydrogenase	Ratio > 0.6 suggests exudative effusion
Protein	Ratio > 0.5 suggests exudative effusion
Glucose	< 40 suggests infection, extremely low levels may be seen with rheumatoid effusions
pH	< 7.2 suggests empyema
Cell count and differential	Polymorphonuclear neutrophil cells most common with bacterial infections, lympho-cytic effusions most common with malignant and tuberculous effusions
Amylase	Elevated with pancreatitis; salivary isoenzymes suggest ruptured esophagus
Triglycerides	Levels > 105 suggest chylothorax
Cholesterol	Elevated levels associated with pseudochylous effusions and exudative effusions
Adenosine deaminase	Elevated levels associated with tuberculous effusions

12

setting of pneumonia of unknown cause, the presence of a lymphocytic exudative effusion should prompt consideration of tuberculosis (TB) or concurrent neoplastic disease.

Tuberculous effusions are usually serous, with total protein > 5.0 g/dL (77% of cases) and with anywhere from 2000 to 8000 nucleated white blood cells (WBC). Most of these WBCs are lymphocytes and in 90% of TB cases more than 60% will be lymphocytes. The exception to this is that early in the course of disease, polymorphonuclear leukocytes may predominate with lymphocytes becoming more common as the disease progresses. Features that make TB less likely include pleural fluid eosinophilia and the presence of more than 5% mesothelial cells. While the measurement of pleural fluid adenosine deaminase, lysozyme and interferon gamma levels may be suggestive, they are not diagnostic of pleural TB.

Unfortunately, the diagnostic yield of acid-fast bacilli (AFB) stain and culture on thoracentesis is also low and therefore the absence of AFB on pleural fluid smear does not exclude TB. Skin testing may be helpful in such cases, since a purified protein derivative (PPD) is positive in 69% to 100% of tuberculous pleural effusions. However, a negative PPD is possible secondary to circulating mononuclear cells that suppress sensitized T lymphocytes in the peripheral blood and skin but do not suppress the inflammation in the pleural space. Similarly, a positive PPD only establishes exposure to TB but does not confirm active disease. Because of the limited utility of pleural fluid smear and culture, the diagnosis of pleural TB is best made by a combination of pleural tissue and fluid histology and culture. The yield of these individual tests is shown in Table 12.3. The combination of these tests as obtained from a closed pleural biopsy establishes the diagnosis of TB in 90% to 95% of cases.

234

TABLE 12.3 — DIAGNOSTIC YIELD OF PROCEDURES IN PLEURAL TUBERCULOSIS

Procedure	Yield (%)
Pleural biopsy histology	60 to 85
Pleural biopsy culture	55 to 80
Pleural fluid culture	13 to 70
Sputum	4 to 50
Pleural biopsy AFB smear	5 to 18
Pleural fluid AFB smear	< 5
Abbreviation: AFB, acid-fast bacilli.	

Assessing the Risk for Complicated Effusions

The importance of pleural fluid analysis in parapneumonic effusions does not lie in the classification of effusions as transudative or exudative. The ultimate goal of pleural fluid analysis is to distinguish those effusions that are most likely to develop into complicated effusions and/or empyema. In addition to pleural fluid analysis, other factors must also be considered in this assessment of risk. These include the virulence of the pathogen as well as host factors. Careful consideration of all of these factors helps determine appropriate interventions.

In the evaluation of most parapneumonic effusions, the most useful diagnostic tests are the pH, LDH, protein, glucose, cell count and Gram stain. In a recent meta-analysis, the pleural fluid pH was found to be the most useful test in determining which parapneumonic effusions should undergo drainage. A pleural pH less than 7.2 represents the threshold for consideration of chest tube drainage. However, other diseases, including malignancy, TB, rheumatoid arthritis, lupus pleuritis and urinothorax may be associated with low pleural pH. Depending upon other concurrent clinical factors, a pH less than 7.2 should prompt consideration of a chest tube. A pH of less than 7.1 strongly supports the need for immediate chest tube drainage.

The pleural fluid LDH, protein, glucose and cell count, while diagnostically useful, are not sufficiently specific to help determine the need for chest tube placement. However, any positive Gram stain should lead to immediate chest tube drainage since this situation is likely to either represent or develop into an empyema. Similarly, if the fluid is grossly purulent, immediate chest tube drainage is warranted.

The virulence of the pathogen must also be considered in assessing the risk for complications. Most commonly, the specific pathogen is unknown at the time of the initial evaluation. If the pathogen is known, however, this may provide additional insight into the likelihood of complications. Organisms such as *Staphylococcus aureus*, gram-negative bacilli and anaerobes are more likely to develop into empyemas. Similarly, although *Streptococcus pneumoniae* is among the most common causes of pneumonia, it rarely develops into actual empyema. In these cases, a more conservative approach may be warranted.

Host factors and preexisting disease also play a significant role in assessing the risk for complications. In the elderly and immunocompromised as well as in those with preexisting lung disease, the spectrum of pathogens causing bacterial pneumonia is significantly different from that in young healthy individuals. The former groups of patients are more likely to have gram-negative pneumonias that are associated with a higher mortality. A more aggressive strategy of intervention may be warranted in this population.

The therapeutic options depend upon the stage of the parapneumonic effusion as well as upon an assessment of the risk of complications developing as described above. In uncomplicated effusions, antibiotics alone are usually sufficient. Serial radiographs are warranted to document improvement of the effusion. Any clinical deterioration or increase in size of the effusion should prompt reevaluation and possibly repeat thoracentesis.

Antibiotic selection in the setting of a parapneumonic effusion should generally be based on the cause of the underlying pneumonia. Consideration should also be given to the possibility of anaerobic infection if there is a particularly large effusion or in the setting of empyema. Since anaerobic organisms are frequently difficult to isolate in clinical laboratories, empiric coverage in this setting may be appropriate. Additional anaerobic coverage can be obtained using clindamycin, metronidazole, β-lactam/β-lactamase combinations, imipenem or trovafloxacin. Almost all antibiotics will penetrate into the pleural space. The one important exception is the inactivation of aminoglycosides at low pleural pH. Thus in the setting of a gram-negative pleural space infection, it is probably warranted to avoid using aminoglycosides as primary therapy.

Complicated parapneumonic effusions are more difficult to manage and tend to have a variable response when treated with antibiotics alone. Although some patients can be managed with antibiotics alone others will develop complications and require chest tube placement. Although there are no prospective clinical trials, there is a bias that early pleural fluid drainage in these cases may improve recovery and decrease length of stay. Certainly those patients with grossly purulent pleural fluid, a positive Gram stain or pleural fluid pH < 7.1 should undergo early drainage. The optimum treatment for patients with exudative effusions with a pH in the intermediate zone of 7.1 to 7.3 is more difficult to determine. Options include early chest tube placement or a trial of antibiotic therapy with a repeat chest radiograph and thoracentesis in 24 to 48 hours to assess response. The choice is often not clear and must include consideration of other factors, including comorbidities and the virulence of the pathogen as described above.

Once the decision has been made that pleural space drainage is needed, there are a number of options available. If the pleural fluid collection is not loculated, then either a large-bore chest tube or a radiographically guided small-bore tube may be used. Importantly, although both methods have been documented to be successful, postdrainage imaging is critical to confirm complete pleural fluid drainage. A high incidence of chest tube failure has been seen when chest tube placement was not followed with adequate imaging and resulted in inadequate drainage.

If the effusion is loculated, treatment options include chest tube placement with intrapleural fibrinolytics and/or thoracoscopy. Intrapleural fibrinolytic therapy consists of regular chest tube placement followed by installation of either 100,000 U urokinase or 250,000 U of streptokinase diluted into 30 to 100 mL of saline. The chest tube is clamped for 2 to 4 hours and then reopened. This is done twice daily until there is resolution of the effusion radiographically. Streptokinase and urokinase appear to be equally effective when used in this fashion, but streptokinase is considerably less costly. Neither regimen induces significant systemic fibrinolysis and thus is relatively safe. Success rates vary in the range of 70% to 90%, although comparative prospective trials are lacking.

Thoracoscopy represents an alternative treatment for loculated effusions. The procedure is somewhat limited by the fact that it can become prolonged if there are extensive adhesions and it is thus best suited for patients with early disease. In those patients that are unable to have adequate drainage or lung re-expansion with thoracoscopy, open decortication may be required. One retrospective series found that up to 30% of empyemas managed with thoracoscopy ultimately required open decortication. Unfortunately, large prospective comparisons are still lacking and thus specific recommendations have not yet been issued regarding the indications for thoracoscopy.

Small case series seem to suggest that thoracoscopy may be superior to intrapleural fibrinolytic therapy. Early thoracoscopy in these series resulted in improved rates of complete pleural drainage, a reduction in chest tube duration and decreased length of stay. A comparison of success rates for the most commonly used procedures is shown in Table 12.4. Importantly, there is a paucity of data directly comparing these procedures, making specific recommendations of limited value.

TABLE 12.4 — SUCCESS RATES FOR PLEURAL DRAINAGE	
Procedure	**Success Rate (%)**
Tube Thoracostomy	
Stage I empyema	70 to 85
Stage II and III empyema	11 to 30
Image-directed catheter drainage	50 to 60
Fibrinolytic therapy	40 to 60
Thoracoscopy	80 to 91
Decortication	90 to 95

Despite adequate drainage procedures, an empyema cavity may fail to resolve. In these cases the empyema cavity often remains because the underlying lung is unable to reexpand because of visceral pleural fibrosis. The thickness of the visceral pleura as well as the size of the cavity determines how likely this is to occur. Those cases that demonstrate failure of pleural apposition after chest tube placement with thickened visceral pleura are candidates for either open thoracostomy or decortication.

Open thoracostomy, while less invasive, is also less effective than open decortication. It is usually preferred to open decortication only in those patients who are too debilitated to withstand open decortication. As such, it is a procedure that is best reserved for debilitated patients who are refractory to management with either fibrinolytics and/or thoracoscopy. Open thoracostomy can be done under local anesthesia and is accomplished by resecting one or more ribs over the lower area of the empyema. A vertical incision through the chest wall then allows open drainage of the empyema cavity. A chest tube is left in place and is gradually withdrawn as the tract closes. This process may take anywhere from 60 to 90 days to complete. Complete healing of the drainage site takes even longer, with a median duration of 142 days in one series.

Decortication represents the most invasive treatment for organized empyema cavities. Typically, this procedure is reserved for those who not only demonstrate pleural thickening but who also remain clinically ill. After allowing the pleural space to organize into a pleural "peel" over a period of several weeks, open resection of the pleural space is undertaken under general anesthesia. All fibrous tissue and purulent material is resected at this time. This procedure is associated with significant perioperative morbidity and is often too difficult for debilitated patients to withstand. In contrast to open thoracostomy drainage, however, open decortication allows a more rapid recovery, with a decreased number of chest tube days and a decreased length of hospital stay.

Summary

Early evaluation of parapneumonic effusions is critical to correctly managing pneumonia. Early thoracentesis should be considered in all patients with significant parapneumonic effusions. The goal of the diagnostic assessment is to identify those effusions that are most likely to develop into complicated effusions or empyemas. A low pH, positive Gram stain or purulent-appearing pleural fluid are all indicators of empyema or complicated effusions and should prompt chest tube placement.

In patients with complicated parapneumonic effusions that are borderline, a trial of antibiotics with repeat thoracentesis may be warranted. Serial radiographs are warranted in all cases to confirm a proper response to drainage. In those patients with effusions that fail to drain or those with loculated effusions, intrapleural fibrinolytic therapy or thoracoscopy may be needed. Finally, in those patients failing fibrinolytic therapy and/or thoracoscopy, open thoracostomy or decortication may be an option. An algorithm summarizing this diagnostic approach is shown in Figure 12.2.

12

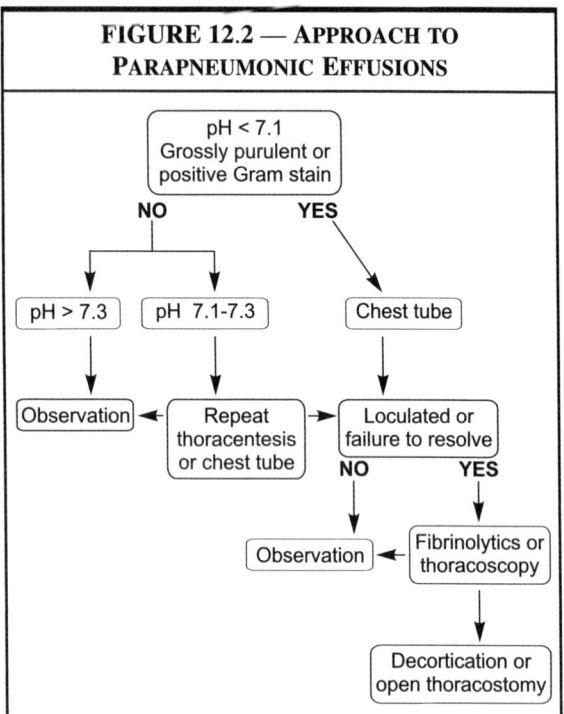

FIGURE 12.2 — APPROACH TO PARAPNEUMONIC EFFUSIONS

pH < 7.1
Grossly purulent or
positive Gram stain

NO   **YES**

pH > 7.3   pH 7.1-7.3   Chest tube

Observation

Repeat thoracentesis or chest tube

Loculated or failure to resolve

NO   **YES**

Observation

Fibrinolytics or thoracoscopy

Decortication or open thoracostomy

SELECTED READINGS

Brook I, Frazier EH. Aerobic and anaerobic microbiology of empyema: a retrospective review of two military hospitals. *Chest*. 1993;103:1502.

Davies CW, Lok S, Davies RJ. The systemic fibrinolytic activity of intrapleural streptokinase. *Am J Respir Crit Care Med*. 1998; 157:328-330.

Fleischner FG. Atypical arrangement of free pleural effusion. *Radiol Clin North Am*. 1963;1:347.

Heffner JE, Brown LK, Barbieri C, DeLeo JM. Pleural fluid chemical analysis in parapneumonic effusions. A meta-analysis [published erratum appears in *Am J Respir Crit Care Med*. 1995;152: 823]. *Am J Respir Crit Care Med*. 1995;151:1700-1708.

Jerjes-Sánchez C, Ramirez-Rivera A, Elizalde JJ, et al. Intrapleural fibrinolysis with streptokinase as an adjunctive treatment in hemothorax and empyema: a multicenter trial. *Chest*. 1996;109:1514-1519.

Kutty CP, Varkey B. "Contarini's condition:" bilateral pleural effusions with markedly different characteristics. *Chest*. 1978;74:679-680.

Lawrence DR, Ohri SK, Moxon RE, Townsend ER, Fountain SW. Thoracoscopic debridement of empyema thoracis. *Ann Thorac Surg*. 1997;64:1448-1450.

LeMense GP, Strange C, Sahn SA. Empyema thoracis. Therapeutic management and outcome. *Chest*. 1995;107:1532-1537.

Light RW, Girard WM, Jenkinson SG, George RB. Parapneumonic effusions. *Am J Med*. 1980;69:507-512.

Müller NL. Imaging of the pleura. *Radiology*. 1993;186:297-309.

Raasch BN, Carsky EW, Lane EJ, O'Callaghan JP, Heitzman ER. Pleural effusion: explanation of some typical appearances. *Am J Roentgenol*. 1982;139:899-904.

Ruskin JA, Gurney JW, Thorsen MK, Goodman LR. Detection of pleural effusions on supine chest radiographs. *Am J Roentgenol*. 1987;148:681-683.

12

Sahn SA. State of the art. The pleura. *Am Rev Respir Dis*. 1988;138:
184-234.

Sahn SA, Light RW. The sun should never set on a parapneumonic
effusion. *Chest*. 1989;95:945-947. Editorial.

Stark DD, Federle MP, Goodman PC, Podrasky AE, Webb WR.
Differentiating lung abscess and empyema: radiography and computed tomography. *Am J Roentgenol*. 1983;141:163-167.

Temes RT, Follis F, Kessler RM, Pett SB Jr, Wernly JA. Intrapleural fibrinolytics in management of empyema thoracis. *Chest*.
1996;110:102-106.

Vaudaux P, Waldvogel FA. Gentamicin inactivation in purulent exu-
dates: role of cell lysis. *J Infect Dis*. 1980;142:586-593.

Wait MA, Sharma S, Hohn J, Dal Nogare A. A randomized trial
of empyema therapy. *Chest*. 1997;111:1548-1551.

Woodring JH. Recognition of pleural effusion on supine radiographs: how much fluid is required? *Am J Roentgenol*. 1984;142:
59-64.

13 Bronchitis

Acute Bronchitis

Acute bronchitis is an inflammatory condition of the tracheobronchial tree that is especially familiar to primary-care physicians. Acute tracheobronchitis is part of a continuum that includes:

- Nasopharyngeal infection
- Bronchitis
- Bronchiolitis
- Pneumonitis.

Symptomatically, these processes may be indistinguishable. Acute tracheobronchitis implies site-specific airway inflammation between the glottis and the bronchioles. In the United Kingdom, 25% of all primary-care visits are related to respiratory disease, and more than half of these are due to upper and lower respiratory tract infections. In 1992, approximately 12 million prescriptions were given for lower respiratory tract infections, accounting for 47.2 million pounds in expenditures. In Europe, more than 80% of all lower respiratory tract infections are treated with antibiotics. Most physicians do not differentiate acute bronchitis, acute exacerbations of chronic bronchitis, community-acquired pneumonia (CAP) and viral respiratory tract infections. The pattern of antibiotic prescribing for these infections varies from country to country, but there is no clear rationale for the antimicrobial choices.

Acute bronchitis occurs most commonly during the winter months when acute respiratory tract infections are prevalent. The mean annual attack rate in the United States for acute bronchitis is approximately 87 cases/100,000 persons/week, peaking in winter at approximately 150 cases/100,000 persons/week. Acute bronchitis accounts for an estimated 12 million physician visits per year, with an annual cost of $200 million to $300 million for physician visits and prescriptions. In a national survey sampling of over 1500 practicing physicians in the United States, 66% of patients with the diagnosis of bronchitis were treated with antibiotics. Risk factors for increased antimicrobial prescribing were female sex and rural practice location, while black race was associated with a lower prescribing rate.

■ Etiology

The syndrome of acute bronchitis is most often associated with respiratory viruses, including common cold viruses (ie, rhinovirus, coronavirus) in addition to more virulent agents such as influenza and adenovirus. Other viral causes of acute bronchitis include measles, respiratory syncytial virus, parainfluenza virus and herpes simplex virus. A small proportion of cases of acute bronchitis are of nonviral etiology. *Mycoplasma pneumoniae, Bordetella pertussis* and *Chlamydia pneumoniae* and TWAR strain are recognized bacterial causes of acute bronchitis. The etiologic role of *Streptococcus pneumoniae* and *Haemophilus influenzae* in acute bronchitis is not clear as these bacteria may represent resident flora of the upper respiratory tract of normal individuals. Acute tracheobronchitis may also be a consequence of the inhalation of irritating, toxic substances as a result of air pollution or occupational exposures, including ammonia, chlorine, sulphur dioxide, nitrogen dioxide and ozone.

■ Pathogenesis

During acute bronchial infection, the mucous membrane of the tracheobronchial tree is hyperemic

246

and edematous. Increased bronchial secretion is also a common feature. While extensive destruction of the respiratory epithelium is seen in infection with influenza, other viral agents such as rhinovirus cause minimal epithelial injury. Impaired mucociliary function is seen in all infections, even in those without overt mucosal damage. Prospective studies frequently fail to isolate a specific pathogen. One explanation may be the delay in seeking medical care after the onset of symptoms, which may bring the patient to medical attention beyond the period of viral shedding. Determination of a causative agent is further complicated in subjects with chronic lung disease who may have tracheobronchial colonization by potentially pathogenic bacteria, including *H influenzae*, *S pneumoniae* and *Moraxella catarrhalis*. A rise in serum antibody titers to bacteria associated with acute bronchitic symptoms suggests that bacteria may play a causative role, although analysis of antibody coating of bacteria in sputum is not helpful.

It is also possible that severity of attacks of acute bronchitis may be increased by exposure to cigarette smoke and air pollutants. These substances, in association with recurrent acute bronchial infection, may result in permanent injury to the bronchial tree. Increased airway reactivity and airway resistance, usually manifested as a bothersome cough, may persist for 6 to 8 weeks. The elevated airway resistance observed after a bronchial infection is largely reversible with β-sympathomimetic and anticholinergic bronchodilators.

■ Clinical Presentation

Cough is uniformly found in acute bronchitis, and it may be productive of mucoid or purulent sputum. The cough may be accompanied by variable amounts of hemoptysis or retrosternal pain that is often described as of a burning quality. It is usually accentuated on inspiration. Generally the temperature is only minimally to moderately elevated. Physical examination often shows harsh breath sounds, rhonchi and variable amounts of expiratory wheezing. Occasionally there are focal areas of diminished breath sounds, which suggest that inspissated mucus has caused atelectasis. Atelectasis may be relieved by the use of humidifiers, bronchodilators, vigorous coughing and, if needed, tracheal suction. Sometimes there is diffuse diminution of air intake or inspiratory stridor. These findings indicate obstruction of major bronchi or the trachea. Most viral acute tracheobronchitis runs a benign, self-limited course. However, herpes simplex type 1 has been associated with severe febrile tracheobronchitis and respiratory failure in normal immunocompetent adults.

■ Diagnosis

Bronchitis may be suspected in patients with an acute respiratory tract infection associated with cough. Bronchitis is a diagnosis of exclusion since many other diseases of the lower respiratory tract can also cause coughing. A complete history should include information on exposure to toxic substances and cigarette use, epidemiologic considerations and vaccination history. A complete physical examination is essential to exclude other causes of cough, including cardiovascular and parenchymal lung disease.

Routine bacterial cultures of expectorated sputum are not helpful because of the sampling problem of contamination by nasopharyngeal flora. Occasionally, the nature of sputum may provide some diagnostic clues. For instance, except for adenovirus infections, the sputum in viral infections almost always shows a marked predominance of mononuclear cells on Gram's or Wright's stain. In contrast, in bacterial infections, the sputum shows a predominance of polymorphonuclear leukocytes. *Mycoplasma* infections are usually associated with mononuclear cells, but there might be a predominant polymorphonuclear cell population. Culture methods and a microimmunofluorescence test have been developed for the laboratory diagnosis of *C pneumoniae*. The use of an immunoglubulin M-(IgM) specific conjugate helps detect current infection. Patients in whom cough persists beyond the expected duration of the acute illness should undergo further diagnostic examination, including chest radiography, sputum cytology and bronchoscopy to exclude other diseases of the tracheobronchial tree and lungs.

■ **Treatment**

In most cases of acute bronchitis, only symptomatic treatment is needed. However, patients with underlying chronic cardiopulmonary disease who contract influenza or other severe forms of bronchitis may develop serious symptoms requiring hospitalization, oxygen therapy and ventilatory assistance. Cough suppressants, adequate hydration to prevent drying of bronchial secretions and symptomatic treatment of mild fever and malaise associated with some influenza syndromes are the cornerstones of treatment of acute bronchitis in otherwise healthy individuals. If bronchospastic symptoms are dominant, there may be a role for inhaled β_2-adrenergic receptor bronchodilators.

The value of antibiotics in the treatment of otherwise healthy individuals with acute bronchitis has not been established and the use of these agents is not recommended as a general practice. This uncertainty stems from conflicting results of clinical trials, which may be explained based on variations in type of antibiotics, dosage schedule, duration of follow-up, the season of the year (reflecting prevalence of different pathogens) and lack of a placebo controlled design in many of these studies. Acute bronchitis caused by *M*

13

pneumoniae infection should be treated with erythromycin or tetracycline; *B pertussis* infection with erythromycin; and *C pneumoniae* infection, with tetracycline, erythromycin or one of the newer macrolide or azalide antibiotics. During epidemics known to be due to influenza A virus, treatment with amantadine is recommended in patients with suspected influenza if the illness is less than 48 hours in duration.

Acute Exacerbations of Chronic Bronchitis

Chronic obstructive pulmonary disease (COPD) afflicts 20% of the population and is the fourth leading cause of death in the Unites States. COPD is a progressive disease characterized by reduced expiratory airflow that is relatively stable over several months of observation. Chronic bronchitis is defined clinically as excessive cough, productive of sputum on most days, for at least 3 months during at least 2 consecutive years.

The major risk factor for chronic bronchitis is cigarette smoking, and cumulative smoking history is most closely related to symptom development. For reasons that are unclear, not all heavy cigarette smokers develop COPD. Familial factors and exposure to dusty environments also play a role, although to a much lesser extent than cigarette smoking. From the Lung Health Study, airways (methacholine) reactivity, after cigarette smoking, was the most important determinant of decline in forced expiratory volume in 1 second (FEV_1). The prognosis of COPD is affected most when lung function as reflected by the FEV_1 falls below 50% of predicted values. When the FEV_1 falls below 1 L, the 5-year survival is approximately 50%.

■ Role of Bacterial Infection

An acute exacerbation of COPD disease is usually defined as an episodic respiratory decompensation without an objectively documented cause such as pneumonia. The role of bacterial infection in acute exacerbation of chronic bronchitis is controversial. Many patients are treated with antibiotics, but the role of antibiotics has been questioned. Several observations have been made in support of bacteria playing an important role. For example, an increased number of bacteria and neutrophils in sputum during exacerbations has been demonstrated. The appearance of an acute antibody response in serum to these bacteria and an increase in inflammatory mediators in purulent sputum suggest a causal relationship. However, the linkage between bacterial infection and symptoms is complicated by a high spontaneous remission rate; this can be expected since bacterial exacerbations are usually limited to the bronchial mucosa.

In a landmark study, Anthonisen and coworkers (1987) demonstrated that patients can be stratified according to symptoms in order to predict a response to antimicrobial therapy. In patients with at least two symptoms, including increased dyspnea, sputum volume and sputum purulence, broad-spectrum antibiotics (amoxicillin, trimethoprim/sulfamethoxazole or doxycycline) led to improved clinical outcomes, fewer therapeutic failures and a more rapid rate of lung function recovery compared to a placebo. Overall, the length of illness was 2 days shorter for the antibiotic-treated group compared with the receiving placebo. If patients presented with three symptoms (type I exacerbation), the difference in outcome for antibiotic-treated patient was greatest, while there was no difference controlled had only one symptom (type III) as for A meta-analysis of nine randomized trials of patients treated for acute exacerbations of chronic

251

bronchitis concluded that a small but statistically significant clinical and physiologic improvement could be expected in antibiotic-treated patients (Table 13.1). A beneficial impact of antibiotics was demonstrated in studies that included the largest number of patients. In the six trials that reported peak expiratory flow rates, an improvement of 10.75 L/min favoring the antibiotic group was noted. While this improvement is small, it may be clinically relevant, particularly in patients with limited respiratory reserve. Design flaws in the earlier studies, such as small number of study patients, unclear selection criteria, uncertain microbiology, nonstandard evaluation criteria and lack of stratification of patients, may account for the discrepancy in outcomes.

Another large randomized, placebo-controlled trial in Italy (Allegra, 1991) has confirmed these operations (Table 13.1). From these considerations, it is apparent that bacterial infection plays a role in a significant proportion of patients experiencing an acute exacerbation of chronic bronchitis, and the use of risk stratification according to the "Anthonisen" criteria will allow the selection of those patients most likely to benefit from antimicrobial therapy.

■ Bacterial Pathogens

Bacterial pathogens can be isolated from sputum in 50% to 60% of patients having an acute exacerbation of chronic bronchitis, with *H influenzae* being the most commonly isolated organism from sputum (Table 13.2). *Haemophilus parainfluenzae, S pneumoniae* and *M catarrhalis* are also found frequently. Studies utilizing the protected specimen brush technique where lower respiratory samples are not contaminated with oropharyngeal samples are not contaminated important role of bacterial have confirmed the tified from pure lower respiratory Organisms identified contaminated by oropharyngeal samples during acute

252

exacerbations are similar (*H influenzae, H parainfluenzae, S pneumoniae, M catarrhalis*) to those found in sputum, but quantitative cultures indicate a greater number of organisms. The number of organisms found in the lower respiratory tract of patients with an acute exacerbation of chronic bronchitis is of the same magnitude seen in patients with ventilator-associated pneumonia, suggesting a considerable bacterial load.

Exacerbations can be caused by endogenous or exogenous reinfection with *H influenzae*. Persistently infected patients keep the same *H influenzae* strain for longer periods, and antibiotic therapy may not be effective in eradicating *H influenzae*. In patients with reasonably well-preserved lung function, gram-positive organisms such as pneumococcus and simple gram-negative organisms such as *H influenzae* and *M catarrhalis* predominate. However, with declining lung function, there is an increasing prevalence of enteric gram-negative organisms and *Pseudomonas aeruginosa*. *H parainfluenzae* has been isolated from sputum in up to 41% of patients with acute exacerbation of chronic bronchitis. Colony counts as high as 9.6×10^8 cfu/mL in sputum cultures and a serum antibody response suggest a potential role for this organism as a true respiratory pathogen. β–Lactamase-mediated amoxicillin resistance is seen in 20% to 40% of *H influenzae* strains in North America and Europe and in almost 100% of *M catarrhalis* strains. In a US survey conducted between 1997 and 1998, 38% of all *H influenzae* isolates were β–lactamase-producing, although a few β–lactamase-negative ampicillin-resistant strains were isolated. In almost 700 strains of *M catarrhalis*, β-lactamase production was found in 92%. In *S pneumoniae*, 25% demonstrated intermediate susceptibility to penicillin, while 12% were penicillin resistant (minimum inhibitory concentration inhibiting 90% of tested strains [MIC_{90}] > 2.0 g/mL).

TABLE 13.1 — OUTCOMES IN ANTIBIOTIC THERAPY FOR EXACERBATION OF CHRONIC OBSTRUCTIVE PULMONARY DISEASE

Comparators	No. of Patients	Outcome of Therapy	Reference
Placebo vs oxytetracycline	37 37	Treated patients lost half as much time from work and exacerbations were shorter	Elmes et al, *BMJ*, 1957.
Placebo vs oxytetracycline	27 26	Treated patients recovered sooner and deteriorated less often	Berry et al, *Lancet*, 1960.
Placebo vs ampicillin	28 28	No significant difference in clinical response	Elmes et al, *BMJ*, 1965.
Placebo vs physiotherapy vs chloramphenicol	10 10 9	No significant differences	Peterson et al, *Acta Med Scand*, 1967.
Placebo vs chloramphenicol vs tetracycline	86 84 89	Antibiotic therapy superior to placebo but no differences between antibiotics	Pines et al, *Br J Dis Chest*, 1972.

Placebo vs tetracycline	20 20	100% vs 100% clinical response	Nicotra et al, *Ann Intern Med*, 1982.
Placebo vs co-trimoxazole, amoxicillin or doxycycline	180 182	55% vs 68% success ($p < 0.01$)	Anthonisen et al, *Ann Intern Med*, 1987.
Placebo vs co-amoxiclav	179 190	50.3% vs 86.4% success ($p < 0.01$)	Allegra et al, *Ital J Chest*, 1991.

From: *Br Med J*. 1957;2:1272-1275, *Lancet*. 1960;1:137-139, *Br Med J*. 1965;2:904-908, *Acta Med Scand*. 1967;182:293-305, *Br J Dis Chest*. 1972;66:107-115, *Ann Intern Med*. 1982;97:18-21, *Ann Intern Med*. 1987;106:196-204, and *Ital J Chest Dis*. 1991;45:138-148.

13

TABLE 13.2 — MICROBIAL ISOLATES IN EXACERBATION OF CHRONIC BRONCHITIS

Study	No. of Isolates	Total Isolates (%)		
		Haemophilus influenzae	*Moraxella catarrhalis*	*Streptococcus pneumoniae*
Davies et al, 1986	127	58.5	15	16.5
Basran et al, 1990	60	43.3	3.3	25
Chodosh, 1992	214	37.9	22.4	22.4
Aldons, 1991	53	70	13	15
Bachand, 1991	84	30	10.7	21.4
Lindsay et al, 1992	398	49.7	19	17
Neu et al, 1993	84	46.4	28.6	25

From: *Pharm Week (sci)*. 1986;8:53-59, *J Antimicrob Chemother*. 1990;26(suppl f):19-24, *Infectious Diseases*. Philadelphia, Pa: WB Saunders Company; 1992:476-485, *J Antimicrob Chemother*. 1991;27(suppl a):101-108, *J Antimicrob Chemother*. 1991;27(suppl a):91-100, *J Antimicrob Chemother*. 1992;30:89-100, and *Chest*. 1993;104:1393-1399.

In a more recent survey conducted between 1994 and 1995 (Doern, 1996), 36.4% of *H influenzae* strains produced β-lactamase. Another 2.5% of *H influenzae* isolates were β-lactamase negative, but ampicillin resistant. β–Lactamase-producing *M catarrhalis* increased to 95.3% of all isolated strains, while the overall frequency of penicillin-resistant *S pneumoniae* increased to 23.6%. Overall, 14.1% of *S pneumoniae* isolates demonstrated intermediate resistance, while 9.5% demonstrated high-level resistance. Of concern was the observation that 9.1% of strains demonstrated multiple-drug resistance. The latest surveys indicate that multidrug-resistant *S pneumoniae* continues to expand, including demonstrating high rates of resistance to macrolides and tetracyclines.

■ Pathogenesis of Bronchial Infections

Cigarette smoking is the most common cause of chronic bronchitis. The mucociliary system forms a primary defense mechanism of the respiratory tract against all inhaled particles, including bacteria. Viral infection and cigarette smoke frequently damage ciliated epithelium, which, in turn, impairs mucociliary clearance. Loss of large areas of ciliated epithelium occurs during viral and bacterial infections and contributes to impaired mucociliary clearance. Delayed mucociliary clearance affords bacteria the opportunity to multiply and attach, first to mucus and then to mucosal surfaces. Organisms such as *H influenzae* produce substances that:

- Impair ciliary function
- Stimulate production of mucus
- Destroy local immunoglobulins
- Impair phagocytic function
- Damage the tracheobronchial epithelium.

H influenzae synthesizes histamine and releases an uncharacterized factor which impairs human neutrophil function. When these bacteria loiter in the airways, a host inflammatory response is stimulated. With the movement of large numbers of neutrophils and their subsequent release of proteinases and toxic oxygen radicals, production of mucus and epithelial surface damage may be enhanced. Progressive airway damage may occur from the products of the bacteria themselves or from the host response to these bacteria. Local host defense may be further impaired, leading to an ever greater chance of bacterial colonization and thus to further damage. This process has been termed the "vicious circle hypothesis" (Figure 2.1) and may account for the insidious progression of airway disease.

■ Risk Stratification

Acute respiratory failure may develop in patients with significant compromise of lung function as a consequence of an acute exacerbation. Identification of these patients and application of an aggressive therapeutic approach from the outset may avoid this important complication. If respiratory failure develops, mechanical ventilation is required in 20% to 60% of patients. Long and expensive intensive-care unit (ICU) hospitalization is common, and hospital mortality rates ranging from 10% to 30% can be expected. Factors reported to be associated with in-hospital mortality include:

- Age > 65 years
- Respiratory dysfunction
- Nonrespiratory organ dysfunction
- Length of hospital stay before ICU admission.

Patient age and severity of airway obstruction in those with COPD have been identified as the major determinants of survival of patients followed for 3 years after discharge from hospital. Other factors linked to survival are performance status and use of oral corticosteroids.

Following institution of antibiotic therapy for an acute exacerbation of chronic bronchitis, factors predicting failure of initial antimicrobial therapy (return to the prescribing physician for more treatment) include coexistent cardiopulmonary diseases and the number of previous exacerbations. The need for hospitalization is best predicted by the presence of significant cardiopulmonary disease. The presence of cardiovascular comorbidity and more than four exacerbations in the previous year has a sensitivity of 70% and specificity of 37% in predicting return to the prescribing physician for further treatment. Advanced age, significant impairment of lung function, poor performance status, comorbid conditions, long duration of chronic bronchitis and a history of previous frequent exacerbations requiring systemic corticosteroid medications characterize a high-risk group of patients.

Since the cost of failure of treatment of these patients is high, an aggressive approach to treatment of this high-risk group might improve outcome. Routine antimicrobial therapy fails in 13% to 25% or more of exacerbations. Therapeutic failure leads to increased cost of care due to extra physician visits, further diagnostic tests and repeated courses of antibiotics. It may also lead to more hospitalizations and prolonged absence from work. Stratification of patients into risk categories may allow the physician to select targeted antimicrobial therapy to prevent some of these consequences. This approach has become increasingly more important due to increasing rates of resistance to standard antimicrobial therapy.

A recent classification divides patients into four groups (Table 13.3). Group 1 patients have tracheobronchitis that is usually viral in origin. Since there is no underlying lung disease in this group, the illness is usually self-limited and runs a benign course.

TABLE 13.3 – CLASSIFICATION OF BRONCHITIS

Baseline Clinical Status	Criteria/Risk Factors	Pathogens	Treatment
I. Acute tracheobronchitis	No underlying structural disease; acute cough and sputum production	Usually viral	None, for prolonged symptoms consider macrolide or tetracycline
II. Simple chronic bronchitis	$FEV_1 > 50\%$, increased sputum volume and purulence, no additional risk factors	*Haemophilus influenzae* *Haemophilus* species *Moraxella catarrhalis* *Streptococcus pneumoniae*	Aminopenicillin Tetracycline Trimethoprim/sulfamethoxazole
III. Complicated chronic bronchitis	Increased sputum volume and purulence + $FEV_1 < 50\%$, advanced age, ≥ 4 exacerbations/y, significant comorbidity, malnutrition, chronic oral steroid usage	As for group II; gram-negatives more likely in patients with $FEV_1 < 50\%$; resistance to β-lactams common	Quinolone β-Lactam/β-lactamase inhibitor Second- or third-generation cephalosporin Second-generation macrolide
IV. Chronic bronchial suppuration	Continuous purulent sputum production with frequent exacerbations	As for group III + Enterobacteriaceae and *Pseudomonas aeruginosa*	Ciprofloxacin or other IV antipseudomonal agents

Abbreviation: FEV_1, forced expiratory volume in 1 second.

Group 2 patients have simple chronic bronchitis, are younger, have only mild-to-moderate impairment of lung function (FEV$_1$ > 50% predicted value) and have less than four exacerbations per year. In this group of patients, typical pathogens, including *H influenzae, S pneumoniae* and *M catarrhalis,* are present, although viral infection often precedes bacterial superinfection. Treatment with a β-lactam is usually successful and the prognosis is excellent. Perhaps this is because many of these patients have a viral infection, and antimicrobial therapy of any kind would be equally successful.

Group 3 patients are older, may have poor underlying lung function (FEV$_1$ < 50% predicted) or only moderate impairment of lung function but have significant comorbidity (diabetes mellitus, congestive heart failure, chronic renal disease, chronic liver disease, etc) and/or experience four or more exacerbations per year. *H influenzae, S pneumoniae* and *M catarrhalis* continue to be the predominant organisms. In patients with more advanced lung disease, gram-negative organisms such as *Klebsiella pneumoniae* or even *P aeruginosa* should be considered. In this group of patients, initial treatment failure has major implications for the patient and health-care system, including increased time lost from work and/or hospitalization. Treatment with medications directed toward resistant organisms, such as a quinolone, amoxicillin-clavulate, second- or third-generation cephalosporins or a second-generation macrolide should perform better than amoxicillin.

Group 4 patients suffer from chronic bronchial suppuration with frequent exacerbations characterized by increased sputum production, increased sputum purulence, cough and worsening dyspnea. Many of these patients will have evidence of bronchiectasis if subjected to high-resolution computed tomography scanning. These individuals tend to have a chronic progressive course, and an aggressive therapeutic approach should be offered. Besides the usual respiratory organisms, other gram-negative organisms, including Enterobacteriaceae and *Pseudomonas* species should be considered as potential pathogens. Ciprofloxacin is the only oral agent with activity against these species and should be considered the agent of choice when they are identified.

■ Nonantimicrobial Treatment

Treatment of acute exacerbation of chronic bronchitis falls into two general approaches of prophylactic and symptomatic therapies.

Preventive Measures

Smoking cessation has been identified as a major cornerstone of management of patients with chronic bronchitis. The recent Lung Health Study confirmed that smoking cessation greatly reduces the rate of decline of FEV_1. The benefit of smoking cessation is seen even among patients over the age of 60. Chronic sputum production often clears within 4 weeks of stopping smoking. Nicotine replacement therapy is an effective approach to smoking cessation, although counseling by a physician has been shown to be the most potent intervention.

Annual influenza vaccination reduces morbidity and mortality of influenza in the elderly by 50%. This beneficial effect is felt to be the result of prevention of airway epithelial damage predisposing to subsequent bacterial infection caused by the virus. The beneficial effect of pneumococcal vaccine in patients with chronic bronchitis has not been firmly established. However, current recommendations are that patients with COPD receive pneumococcal vaccine (Pneumovax) at least once in their life and consideration be given to repeating the vaccine every 5 to 10 years, especially in high-risk patients or those that have a rapid decline in pneumococcal antibody levels.

Symptomatic Therapy

Generally, a combination of inhaled anticholinergic with inhaled β-agonist is used in treatment of acute exacerbation of chronic bronchitis. The method of delivery of inhaled bronchodilators has not been shown to influence clinically significant outcomes. The long-term administration of inhaled anticholinergics does not alter the prognosis of COPD. Aminophylline in acute exacerbation of chronic bronchitis adds little to the bronchodilating potential of inhaled medications and increases side effects. Oxygen therapy to maintain a PO_2 above 60 mm Hg or an arterial oxygen saturation more than 90% may be required. Excessive use of oxygen should be avoided as this may lead to progressive hypercapnia, either by decreasing hypoxic ventilatory drive or by worsening ventilation-perfusion mismatching within the lung.

Retrospective reviews of patients presenting to the emergency department with acute exacerbation of COPD show a clear benefit in the group treated with corticosteroids. Faster improvement of pulmonary function tests utilizing parenteral corticosteroids during acute exacerbations of COPD has been reported. The results of the current Systemic Corticosteroids in COPD Exacerbation (SCCOPE) clinical trial being conducted by the Veterans' Affair in the United States suggest a role for oral corticosteroids. Currently, the weight of clinical evidence supports use of a course of systemic corticosteroids in the management of acute exacerbation of chronic bronchitis.

13

SUGGESTED READINGS

Aldos PM. A comparison of clarithromycin with ampicillin in the treatment of outpatients with acute bacterial exacerbation of chronic bronchitis. *J Antimicrob Chemother.* 1991;27(suppl a):101-108.

Allegra L, Grassi C, Grossi E, Pozzi E. Ruolo degli antibiotici nel trattamento della riacutizza della bronchite cronica. *Ital J Chest Dis.* 1991;45:138-148.

American Thoracic Society. Standards for the diagnosis and care of patients with chronic obstructive pulmonary disease (COPD) and asthma. *Am Rev Respir Dis.* 1987;136:225-244.

Anthonisen NR, Connett JE, Kiley JP, et al. Effects of smoking intervention and the use of an inhaled anticholinergic bronchodilator on the rate of decline of FEV1. The Lung Health Study. *JAMA.* 1994;272:1497-1505.

Anthonisen NR, Manfreda J, Warren CP, Hershfield ES, Harding GK, Nelson NA. Antibiotic therapy in exacerbations of chronic obstructive pulmonary disease. *Ann Intern Med.* 1987;106:196-204.

Bachand RT. Comparative study of clarithromycin and ampicillin in the treatment of patients with acute bacterial exacerbations of chronic bronchitis. *J Antimicrob Chemother.* 1991;27(suppl 1):91-100.

Ball P, Harris JM, Lowson D, Tillotson G, Wilson R. Acute infective exacerbations of chronic bronchitis. *Q J Med.* 1995;88:61-68.

Basran GS, Joseph J, Abbas AM, Hughes C, Rotherham UK. Treatment of acute exacerbations of chronic obstructive airways disease: a comparison of amoxycillin and ciprofloxacin. *J Antimicrob Chemother.* 1990;26(suppl 5):19-24.

Berry DG, Fry J, Hindley CP, et al. Exacerbations of chronic bronchitis treatment with oxytetracycline. *Lancet.* 1960;1:137-139.

Butler JC, Breinan RF, et al. Pneumococcal polysaccharide vaccine efficacy: an evaluation of current recommendation. *JAMA.* 1993; 270:1826-1831.

Boldy DA, Skidmore SJ, Ayres JG. Acute bronchitis in the community: clinical features, infective factors, changes in pulmonary function and bronchial reactivity to histamine. *Respir Med.* 1990; 84:377-385.

Chodosh S. Bronchitis and asthma. In: Gorbach SL, Bartlett JG, Blacklow NR, eds. *Infectious Diseases*. Philadelphia, Pa: WB Saunders Company; 1992:476-485.

Cole P, Wilson R. Host-microbial interrelationships in respiratory infection. *Chest*. 1989;95(suppl):217S-221S.

Davies TI, Maesen FPV, Teengs JP, Baur C. The quinolones in chronic bronchitis. *Pharm Week (sci)*. 1986;8:53-59.

Derenne JP, Fleury B, Pariente R. Acute respiratory failure of chronic obstructive pulmonary disease. *Am Rev Respir Dis*. 1988; 138:1006-1033.

Doern GV, Brueggemann A, Holley HP Jr, Rauch AM. Antimicrobial resistance of *Streptococcus pneumoniae* recovered from outpatients in the United States during the winter months of 1994 to 1995: results of a 30-center national surveillance study. *Antimicrob Agents Chemother*. 1996;40:1208-1213.

Elmes PC, Fletcher CM, Dutton AAC. Prophylactic use of oxytetracycline for exacerbations of chronic bronchitis. *Br Med J*. 1957;2:1272-1275.

Elmes PC, King TKC, Langlands JHM, et al. Value of ampicillin in the hospital treatment of exacerbations of chronic bronchitis. *Br Med J*. 1965;2:904-908.

Eller J, Ede A, Schaberg T, Niederman MS, Mauch H, Lode H. Infective exacerbations of chronic bronchitis: relation between bacteriologic etiology and lung function. *Chest*. 1998;113:1542-1548.

Fagon JY, Chastre J, Trouillet JL, et al. Characterization of distal bronchial microflora during acute exacerbation of chronic bronchitis. Use of the protected specimen brush technique in 54 mechanically ventilated patients. *Am Rev Respir Dis*. 1990;142:1004-1008.

Gonzales R, Steiner JF, Sande MA. Antibiotic prescribing for adults with colds, upper respiratory tract infections, and bronchitis by ambulatory care physicians. *JAMA*. 1997;278:901-904.

Grossman RF. Guidelines for the treatment of acute exacerbations of chronic bronchitis. *Chest*. 1997;112(suppl 6):310S-313S.

Gump DW, Phillips CA, Forsyth BR, McIntosh K, Lamborn KR, Stouch WH. Role of infection in chronic bronchitis. *Am Rev Respir Dis*. 1976;113:465-474.

13

Lindsay G, Scorer HJ, Carnegie CM. Safety and efficacy of temafloxacin versus ciprofloxacin in lower respiratory tract infections: a randomized, double-blind trial. *J Antimicrob Chemother.* 1992;30:89-100.

Monsó E, Ruiz J, Rosell A, et al. Bacterial infection in chronic obstructive pulmonary disease. A study of stable and exacerbated outpatients using the protected specimen brush. *Am J Respir Crit Care Med.* 1995;152(pt 1):1316-1320.

Morrell DC. Expressions of morbidity in general practice. *Br Med J.* 1971;2:454-458.

Murphy TF, Sethi S. Bacterial infection in chronic obstructive pulmonary disease. *Am Rev Respir Dis.* 1992;146:1067-1083.

Neu HC, Chick TW. Efficacy and safety of clarithromycin compared to cefixine as outpatient treatment of lower respiratory tract infections. *Chest.* 1993;104:1393-1399.

Nicotra MB, Rivera M, Awe RJ. Antibiotic therapy of acute exacerbations of chronic bronchitis. A controlled study using tetracycline. *Ann Intern Med.* 1982;97:18-31.

Peterson ES, Esmann V, Honcke P, Munkner C. A controlled study of the effect of treatment on chronic bronchitis. An evaluation using pulmonary function tests. *Acta Med Scand.* 1967;182:293-305.

Pines A, Raafat H, Greenfield JS, Linsell WD, Solari ME. Antibiotic regimens in moderately ill patients with purulent exacerbations of chronic bronchitis. *Br J Dis Chest.* 1972;66:107-115.

Saint S, Bent S, Vittinghoff E, Grady D. Antibiotics in chronic obstructive pulmonary disease exacerbations. A meta-analysis. *JAMA.* 1995;273:957-960.

Seneff MG, Wagner DP, Wagner RP, Zimmerman JE, Knaus WA. Hospital and 1-year survival of patients admitted to intensive care units with acute exacerbation of chronic obstructive pulmonary disease. *JAMA.* 1995;274:1852-1857.

INDEX

Note: Page numbers in *italics* indicate figures;
page numbers followed by t indicate tables.

14

267

14

270

14

271

14

14

14

14

14

14

14

14